Good Clinical Practices in Pharmaceuticals

Good clinical practice (GCP) is a set of internationally recognized ethical and scientific quality requirements that must be followed when designing, conducting, recording, and reporting trials that involve the participation of human subjects. Compliance with GCP assures patients and the public that the rights, safety, and wellbeing of people taking part in studies are protected and that research data is reliable.

1. Presents details on GCP, the international ethical, scientific, and practical standard to which all clinical research is conducted.
2. Provides the most up-to-date and best practices, techniques, and methodologies in good clinical practice.
3. Discusses applicable laws and regulations supporting GCP compliance, quality and operations.
4. Describes who is responsible for implementing and maintaining quality assurance and quality control systems to ensure that studies are conducted and data are generated, documented, and reported in compliance with the protocol.

Drugs and the Pharmaceutical Sciences
A Series of Textbooks and Monographs

Series Editor
Anthony J. Hickey
RTI International, Research Triangle Park, USA

The Drugs and Pharmaceutical Sciences series is designed to enable the pharmaceutical scientist to stay abreast of the changing trends, advances and innovations associated with therapeutic drugs and that area of expertise and interest that has come to be known as the pharmaceutical sciences. The body of knowledge that those working in the pharmaceutical environment have to work with, and master, has been, and continues, to expand at a rapid pace as new scientific approaches, technologies, instrumentations, clinical advances, economic factors and social needs arise and influence the discovery, development, manufacture, commercialization and clinical use of new agents and devices.

RNA-seq in Drug Discovery and Development
Feng Cheng and Robert Morris

Patient Safety in Developing Countries: Education, Research, Case Studies
Yaser Al-Worafi

Industrial Hygiene in the Pharmaceutical and Consumer Healthcare Industries
Casey Cosner

Cancer Targeting Therapies: Conventional and Advanced Perspectives
Muhammad Yasir Ali, Shazia Bukhari

Molecular Recognition in Pharmacology
Mikhail Darkhovskiy

GMP Audits in Pharmaceutical and Biotechnology Industries
Mustafa EDİK

Purification of Biotechnological Products: A Focus on Industrial Applications
Adalberto Pessoa Jr, Beatriz Vahan Kilikian and Paul Long

Principles of Research Methodology and Ethics in Pharmaceutical Sciences: An Application Guide for Students and Researchers
Vikas Anand Saharan, Hitesh Kulhari, and Hemant Jadhav

Good Clinical Practices in Pharmaceuticals
Graham P. Bunn

For more information about this series, please visit: www.crcpress.com/Drugs-and-the-Pharmaceutical-Sciences/book-series/IHCDRUPHASCI

Good Clinical Practices in Pharmaceuticals

Edited by
Graham P. Bunn

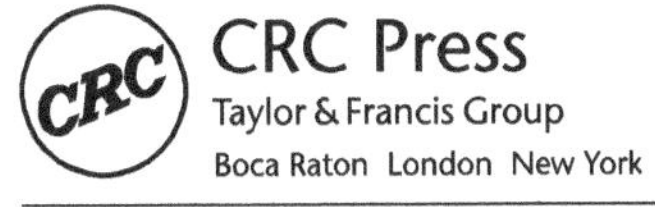

CRC Press is an imprint of the
Taylor & Francis Group, an **informa** business

Designed cover image: Shutterstock

First edition published 2025
by CRC Press
2385 Executive Center Drive, Suite 320, Boca Raton, FL 33431

and by CRC Press
4 Park Square, Milton Park, Abingdon, Oxon, OX14 4RN

CRC Press is an imprint of Taylor & Francis Group, LLC

Library of Congress Cataloging-in-Publication Data
Names: Bunn, Graham P., editor.
Title: Good clinical practices in pharmaceuticals / edited by Graham P. Bunn.
Other titles: Drugs and the pharmaceutical sciences 0360-2583
Description: First edition. | Boca Raton, FL : CRC Press, 2025. |
Series: Drugs and the pharmaceutical sciences | Includes bibliographical references and index.
Identifiers: LCCN 2024023521 | ISBN 9781032524078 (hardback) |
ISBN 9781032525259 (paperback) | ISBN 9781003407010 (ebook)
Subjects: MESH: Clinical Trials as Topic–standards | Drug Evaluation–standards |
Human Experimentation–standards | Legislation as Topic | United States
Classification: LCC R853.C55 | NLM QV 771.4 | DDC 615.5072/4–dc23/eng/20240705
LC record available at https://lccn.loc.gov/2024023521

ISBN: 9781032524078 (hbk)
ISBN: 9781032525259 (pbk)
ISBN: 9781003407010 (ebk)

DOI: 10.1201/9781003407010

Typeset in Times
by codeMantra

Contents

Preface

Welcome to an extensive knowledge resource of Good Clinical Practices worldwide guidance and requirements. I am in debt to the contributing authors who bring many years of expertise, have taken time from their busy schedules to share this with you, the reader, and are passionate about what they do. The insight into protecting patient safety in clinical research does not get any closer to patients than this book. A very personal experience in the introduction will compel you to read the first-hand knowledge and best practices from decades of experience. Everyone is driven by the daily reminder, 'patients first today and every day'. Patients are why we do this because we do what we love and love what we do 'with passion', each and every day.

Graham P. Bunn

Editor

Graham P. Bunn has been the president of GB Consulting LLC, in Pennsylvania, since 2000 and provides regulatory compliance guidance and technical consulting services for pharmaceutical, biotechnology, and other FDA-related industries. His experience includes supporting and leading teams for quality systems assessments, regulatory action responses and remediations (FDA483, Warning Letter, Consent Decree), and preparing sites to host regulatory inspections. He has developed and facilitated numerous highly interactive learning workshops worldwide, including Aseptic Training Programs, Batch Record Reviews, QA on the Floor, and aseptic training support for Compounding Centers. Before founding GB Consulting LLC, Graham gained extensive experience through various management positions in the pharmaceutical industry with SmithKline Beecham PLC (GlaxoSmithKline PLC), Wyeth Pharmaceuticals (Pfizer), and Astra Merck Inc. (AstraZeneca PLC). His career includes management responsibilities as a corporate compliance auditor, quality assurance, validation, and clinical trials manufacturing and packaging. Graham is the editor of Good Manufacturing Practices for Pharmaceuticals and Good Laboratory Practices for Non-Clinical Studies and the author of several book chapters/journal articles. Graham received a BSc in pharmacy from Brighton University, England, and an MSc in Quality Assurance and Regulatory Affairs from Temple University, Philadelphia, and is a member of the Regulatory Affairs Professional Society (RAPS).

Contributors

Randall Basinger
Principal Consultant and Founder, Common Sense Validation Consultants, LLC

Dr. Graham Bunn
eClinical Edge LTD
Reading, United Kingdom

Jessica Chu
CandorVigilance Pte. Ltd.
Singapore

Sonya T. Edgerton
Conformity Compliance Consultants, LLC
Lydbrook, England

Aurea Flores
Aurea Flores Consultants, LLC
Scottsdale, AZ, USA

Connie Freund
Stremline Theraputics, Inc.
New York, New York

Shanthi Ganeshan
Stremline Theraputics, Inc.
New York, New York

Glenda Guest
Assured of Quality Consulting & Training
Flagstaff, Arizona

John S. Klein
NorthCoast Clinical Consulting, LLC
Cleveland, Ohio

Jennifer Lawyer
Clinical Pathways
Cary, NC USA

Tommy Lee
MSHS
Shady Shores, Texas

Joseph Near
J Charles Consulting
Holly Springs, North Carolina

Arthur Ooghe
Cognivia S.A.
Mont-Saint-Guibert, Belgium

Sandra "Sam" Sather
Clinical Pathways LLC
Chapel Hill, North Carolina

Vaska Tone
LaVaPharm LLC
Sheridan, Wyoming

Karen Truhe
Sláinte Consulting, LLC
Waretown, New Jersey

Introduction

Welcome to the world of Good Clinical Practices (GCP) and the relevant connections that play a large part in how human clinical trials and eventually the medicines and devices are regulated, managed, and completed with the thought of bringing to market effective and safe products to the consumer. Unfortunately, we all know of at least one skeptic that talks about Big Pharma and the suppression of "cures" for any and all aliments from Covid to Cancer, from Alzheimer's to Zika Virus. Realistically, there are just too many moving parts within a pharmaceutical, biotechnology, or device company to ever warrant that any CEO has a final say as to what gets developed and ultimately to the patient and what gets stockpiled for future use or left on the shelf. As for cures, well, those would be the most profitable as a one-time solution worth millions to some and not affordable to others, but how realistic is it really? Do you really think that the ultra-rich would not be able to get their hands on a "cure" if one existed, someone like Steve Jobs, the co-founder of Apple, who died of pancreatic cancer, or Colin Powel, the first black Secretary of State in the USA, who died of Covid?

For those of us contributing our knowledge of GCP to this book, we can easily say that we have worked on, contributed to, audited, and been inspected by too many people and regulators to even so much as acknowledge a whim that there is any truth to Big Pharma myths. We all have loved ones who have benefited from the products that have made it to the pharmacy dispensary years or even decades after discovery in the laboratory. One of the biggest reasons that the authors of this book are contributing their time and energy even when we have our own busy lives to attend to is the fact that those loved ones mean a lot to us, as they do to you, the reader. So, let's bring this whole clinical trial and good clinical practices topic into a better perspective for you.

I am a pharmaceutical professional who has worked in various positions within various companies in my 30+ year career. I worked in the research laboratory, where we did chemistry and analyzed potential new molecular entities. I worked in the toxicology laboratory, where we tested whether the drug we had just discovered and made up from scratch in the chemistry lab might work on a living organism. I worked in data management and statistics, where we developed methods to figure out whether our medicine worked against a placebo or against another product already marketed and to see if our medicine was perhaps more effective or was safer than what was already available to patients. My final and most beloved position is my profession as an auditor, where I perform reviews of data, people, and processes to ensure that we all keep it honest from beginning to end and comply with federal and international requirements.

I have seen the evolution of a medicine from the research laboratory, through the clinical trial testing phase, to the statistical analysis of millions of data points, to applying for marketing approvals, and finally to post-marketing safety. The majority of my career has been spent working and auditing in the area of cancer research. I have worked for countless hours on endless clinical trials involving numerous types of cancer. You name it, I probably worked on it. I've worked on chemotherapies, immunotherapies, vaccines, CAR-T therapies, and patient-named projects. I've traveled to 48 of the 50 United States, to over 25 countries, and to hospitals and private clinics around the globe. Nice for me, right? Well, let me bring all of this experience into perspective.

Let me take you to my most dear and most difficult route to this introduction, my daughter. You see, my daughter at the age of 18 was diagnosed with one of the rarest forms of pediatric cancer, called Ewing Sarcoma. Even though I had years of cancer trial experience, I learned that the treatment options for my daughter's cancer had not changed in over 40 years, and very few pharmaceutical companies had any plans or trials that I could get my daughter on. Naturally, we started with the 40-year-old treatment. In the meantime, with my connections and clinical trial experience, I called, texted, emailed, video-conferenced with every pharmaceutical and biotechnology company working on any Ewing Sarcoma clinical trial, or any oncologist who had any access to any clinical trial. In the end, we actually got the same attention and priority as any other patient who qualified to participate in a clinical trial, which made us really appreciate that we are all important and that no one is more important than another.

Clinical trials offer the patient the opportunity to participate in the most recent, up-to-date research on the planet. The companies and the people that put together the trials aren't just pushing something "discovered" in the laboratory; in fact, the amount of research and references to other scientists' research is reams of peer-reviewed medical journal articles. The protocols have to be reviewed and approved by committees for both research and ethics. The trials have to be reviewed and approved by regulatory bodies in each country before they are open to patients. Any changes need to be approved before they can be implemented. The trials must have a data safety monitoring board to make sure that the product remains safe and effective for the full time that the trial is ongoing, and if any of these fail, the trial is shut down. What more could I do as a pharmaceutical professional, or better yet, as a mother who loves her daughter unconditionally but wants to get her participation in a clinical trial? Unfortunately, my daughter passed away even though we had put her on immunotherapy and had just gotten her onto a CAR-T treatment, but her cancer was faster than her immune system.

I took a year off to mourn, but I am not discouraged that there will be a cure someday for many diseases, if not for all cancer types or for all diseases, but for new discoveries. There will be medicinal products for diseases that are "mainstream", like Type II diabetes, or "orphan" drugs for those very rare, one-in-a million diseases that only a few patients need. The most significant course of any product making it onto the market for sale and approved by a regulatory agency like the US Food and Drug Administration (FDA) or the European Medicines Agency (EMA) is that every pharmaceutical, biotechnology, or device company must comply with Good Clinical Practices. It's the peace of mind that all participants can rest assured of and that we count on as people and patients.

I will leave it to you, the reader, to get to know what GCP entails, what it "is all about", and the various aspects of clinical trials, including relevant regulations, quality, consents, data, inspections, and approvals, before any medicine or device ever makes it into your hands.

Vaska Tone
CEO at LaVaPharm LLC

1 FDA Submission Requirements

Shanthi Ganeshan and Connie Freund

GCP FRAMEWORK

In 1996, the International Conference on Harmonization of Technical Requirements for Registration of Pharmaceuticals for Human Use (ICH) developed "*Guidance for Industry Good Clinical Practice (ICH GCP E6 (R2))*" [1]. This provides a unified standard for many countries, including the European Union (EU), Canada, Japan, and the United States, to comply with the regulatory authorities. It is also recognized globally for its framework of rigor and expectations regarding clinical trial conduct and evaluations, and many countries utilize ICH guidance, ensuring GCPs along the way.

The principles of GCP help assure the safety, integrity, and quality of clinical trials by addressing elements related to the design, conduct, and reporting of these trials. GCP training describes the responsibilities of investigators, sponsors, monitors, and IRBs in the conduct of clinical trials [2].

GCP training helps to ensure the following:

- The rights, safety, and well-being of human trial participants are protected.
- Clinical trials are conducted in accordance with approved plans.
- Data generated from clinical trials are reliable.

GCPs are at the heart of drug development. In industry, at the heart of drug development is true cross-functional collaboration. Global Regulatory Affairs is one aspect of that cross-functional collaboration in any organization.

Global Regulatory Affairs: A Key Development Partner

The Global Regulatory Affairs (GRA) professional in the sponsor's organization is typically responsible for facilitating regulatory approvals for new pharmaceutical products, ensuring that the approved products are compliant with local regulations so they can be maintained on the market (for example, fulfilling post-marketing reporting requirements and commitments to health authorities).

GRA professionals, working as part of a product team, develop regulatory strategies to enable pathways to innovative medicines for patients. To do this, the GRA professional evaluates challenges, identifies risks, and develops mitigation approaches with the development team of cross-functional subject matter experts (SMEs). Providing this strategic direction to product development, participating in

DOI: 10.1201/9781003407010-1

discussions on innovative science, and helping to ensure compliance requirements are met are also key activities for the GRA professional.

General regulatory objectives include the following activities* (not exhaustive):

- Creation of development and registration goals by devising a regulatory strategy and collaborating to drive its execution.
- Maintenance of knowledge of changing pharmaceutical legislation.
- Preparation and submission of registration documents to regulatory agencies.
- Providing strategic and technical/regulatory advice throughout product development, including the preparation of regulatory dossiers for investigational products and submission for marketing authorization applications. *Relevant parts of GCPs will be expanded in subsequent chapters of this book.

One of the important responsibilities of the GRA professional is to be the sponsor's main point of contact with Regulatory Authorities, such as the United States (US) Food and Drug Administration (FDA).

For simplicity purposes, this chapter will be centered on the US FDA policies, procedures, and application requirements, with a focus on how GCPs integrate into all these activities for a sponsor.

Where relevant, the comparable global aspects of applications and regulatory processes will be highlighted.

The first section provides an overview of the FDA and its structure and regulations of interest within the Pharmaceutical Industry.

OVERVIEW OF THE US FDA

The FDA is responsible for protecting public health by ensuring the safety, efficacy, and security of human and veterinary drugs, biological and vaccine products, medical devices, food, tobacco, cosmetics, and products that emit radiation. The FDA also provides accurate, science-based health information to the public [3]. The FDA is headquartered in Silver Spring, Maryland, and its current Commissioner and organizational structure can be found on its website [4]. The Administration is broken down into various divisions, and for the purposes of GCPs, the focus will be on the Center for Drug Evaluation and Research (CDER) and the Center for Biologics Evaluation and Research (CBER). CDER is comprised of various offices; the Office of New Drugs (OND) within CDER (further separated into different therapeutic areas, such as Cardiology, Respiratory, Neurology, and Oncology, to name a few) is the main Agency within CDER, reviewing the sponsor submissions and application requirements that are highlighted in the subsequent sections of this chapter. For CBER, the regulation and review of applications pertaining to biological and related products, including blood, vaccines, allergens, tissues, and cellular and gene therapies, is its focus.

Food, Drug & Cosmetic Act

As per the FDA, the Food, Drug & Cosmetic Act (FD&C) is the

> basic food and drug law of the U.S. The law is intended to assure consumers that foods are pure and wholesome, safe to eat, and produced under sanitary conditions; that drugs and devices are safe and effective for their intended uses; that cosmetics are safe and made from appropriate ingredients; and that all labeling and packaging is truthful, informative, and not deceptive [5].

Historically, what has now become the FDA as an institution has evolved over time, but the most notable change to the FDA remit in modern history can be traced back to a therapeutic disaster that occurred in 1937: Elixir Sulfanilamide.

Over 100 people died, including many children, due to untested ingredients (toxic diethylene glycol instead of glycerol) being used in the product. As per the FDA

> the public outcry not only reshaped the drug provisions of the new law to prevent such an event from happening again, it propelled the bill itself through Congress. FDR signed the Food, Drug, and Cosmetic Act on 25 June 1938.
>
> *(Part II: 1938, Food, Drug, Cosmetic Act [6])*

Under the FD&C Act, the FDA has broad authority to regulate drugs, including clinical testing, approval, safety, manufacturing, reporting, distribution, advertising, promotions, sales, imports, and exports. Additional amendments to the FD&C Act have been introduced throughout the years.

Section 505 of the FD&C Act "prohibits traffic of new drugs unless such drugs have been adequately tested to show that they are safe for use under the conditions of use prescribed in their labeling. FDA may authorize exemption from this requirement for drugs intended solely for investigational use by qualified scientific experts".

In addition, it is also stated that "the secretary shall promulgate regulations for exempting from the foregoing subsections for drugs intended solely for investigational use by experts qualified by scientific training and experience to investigate the safety and efficacy of drugs".

Hence, the FDA oversees all aspects of investigational new drug (IND pre-market approval), new drug applications (NDA/BLA), abbreviated new drug applications (ANDA) reviews, and safety surveillance for drugs in development and available on the market.

US Code of Federal Regulations

Since this chapter and book refer to several US Code of Federal Regulations (CFR), an overview of the CFR is outlined.

The CFR is defined as "*a codification (arrangement of) the general and permanent rules published in the Federal Register by the executive departments and agencies of the Federal Government*" [7].

It is published annually and is divided into 50 titles that represent areas that are under the remit of federal regulations. Each of the 50 titles contains various volumes. While working within GCPs, there are specific CFR parts and subparts that should be highlighted for any organization to comply with. While many will be cited throughout this book, the focus of this chapter is on the two sections most commonly of interest to pharmaceutical organizations:

- 21 CFR 312: Investigational New Drug Application
- 21 CFR 314: Applications for FDA Approval to Market New Drugs

Working with FDA

The FDA's guiding principle is its mission to promote and protect public health. For new drugs and products, it accomplishes this during product development through the Investigational New Drug or IND stage, during the review of a New Drug Application (NDA – see Section *"NDA process and Lifecyle Management"*), and subsequently, after NDA approval, through the continued safety monitoring of that product.

The NDA is typically used for drugs that are classified as new chemical entities or small molecules. A Biologics License Application (BLA) is the equivalent application for biologics, with certain differences (refer to 21 CFR 601 for specifics). In Europe and other ex-US regions, the equivalent is often referred to as a Marketing Authorization Application (MAA).

This chapter will focus on the NDA process.

A typical product lifecycle is presented in Figure 1.1.

Please note that Figure 1.1 is not representative of development timelines and corresponding stages.

FDA Meetings

Highlighting the key roles of the company/organization's GRA representative and the entire cross-functional product team, a sponsor's dialogue and interaction with the FDA for a specific molecule or product's development program can span

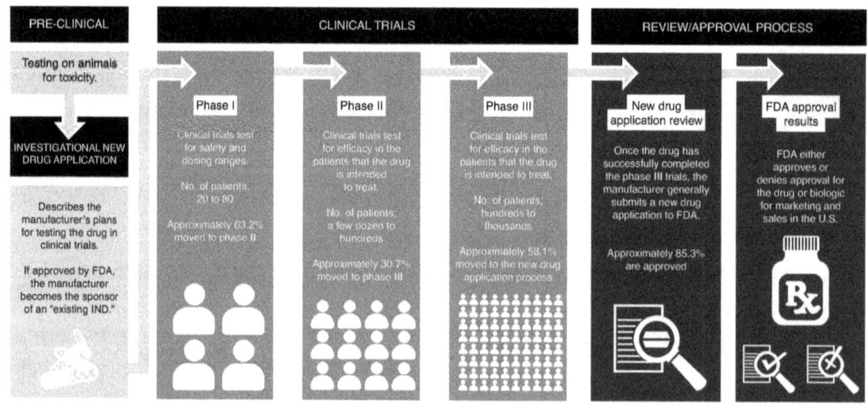

FIGURE 1.1 Example of typical product lifecycle.

Source: GAO analysis of FDA data and a 2016 collaborative study by Biotechnology Innovation Organization, Biomedtracker and Amplion.

approximately 5–10 years or longer before the NDA can be supported for submission and potential approval of a new molecular or chemical entity (NME/NCE).

These interactions with the FDA are typically facilitated through formal meetings with the sponsor and agency and via FDA feedback provided via certain IND submissions [8]. The meeting format can be "written feedback only", teleconference, or Face-to-Face (in person or virtually). With any meeting, a written meeting request, followed by a meeting briefing package, is required to both secure the meeting with appropriate FDA experts, facilitate the meeting discussion, and solicit the agency's feedback on topics raised by the sponsor.

The FDA's experts will provide feedback on the sponsor's proposed topics for the specific meeting and often include the agency's representatives, such as the Division Director, Medical Officer, Clinical Pharmacologist, Statistical Team Leader, Safety Team Leader, Regulatory Project Manager, and Toxicology Team Leader.

For brevity, the typical meetings available to a sponsor with the FDA are described below. Please note that the FDA may request discussions with the sponsor at any time during the drug development lifecycle, at their discretion.

Type A Meeting

- Often reserved for what are deemed critical issues so that the sponsor and FDA can work on a path forward for aspects that might otherwise stall development. These aspects may include meetings to resolve clinical holds or special protocol assessments, urgent safety aspects, etc.
- Has the most expedited timeline of FDA meetings:
  - scheduled to occur within 30 days of the request; thus, the meeting request and briefing package are often submitted together (per current FDA Guidance, the briefing package is due 14 days before the granted meeting date).

Type B Meetings

- Usually held as needed for the categories of preIND and preNDA meetings.
  - Scheduled to occur within 60 days of the meeting request.
- Type B meetings are further subdivided into an additional category referred to as End-of-Phase (EOP) Meetings. These EOP Meetings are held as deemed necessary by the sponsor for EOP1 and EOP2 and abide by a different set of timelines than standard type B meetings described above.
  - Scheduled to occur within 70 days of the meeting request.

Type C Meetings

- A Type C meeting is any meeting other than a Type A, Type B, or Type B (EOP) scheduled to discuss certain aspects of a product.
  - Scheduled to occur within 75 days of the meeting request.

Please note that new additional categories of meetings are available with the FDA and can be found in further detail in the Draft Guidance for Industry Sep. 2023 [8].

Equivalent interactions and opportunities with ex-US regulatory agencies are also available during the product's development, depending on the sponsor's regulatory strategy. An example is EU Scientific Advice [9].

IND APPLICATION PROCESS AND LIFECYCLE MANAGEMENT

IND Application: FDA Requirements and Process

Types of INDs and Categories of INDs

The IND is the primary mechanism to obtain a legal exemption from federal statutes, which highlight that an investigational drug cannot be shipped across state lines for clinical evaluations in humans [10]. Overall, the purpose of the IND is to provide the data, scientific rationale, and evidence to support the evaluation of the investigational product in human clinical trial participants.

In general, there are two main categories of INDs: Noncommercial and Commercial.

Noncommercial INDs are often submitted by organizations or physicians with a goal that is generally not commercial in nature. This could be a physician wanting to evaluate a drug's effects in one or more of their patients (referred to as an "investigator-initiated IND) or an organization/company's intent to use a product under emergency use, which may be directed by a public health crisis such as Covid-19.

For the purposes of brevity, this regulatory chapter focuses on aspects of **Commercial INDs**, which are the most common types of INDs within the pharmaceutical/biotech industry and are filed by companies that want to initiate Phase I (and Phase 2 and 3) trials in the US with the ultimate goal of seeking approval of that drug for use in an intended patient population.

What is an IND (21 CFR 312.22)?

Before a new drug or biologic is made available via prescription to patients (marketed product), it needs to be evaluated for safety and effectiveness in a proposed indication or therapeutic area. This is usually accomplished by the characterization of the molecule via in vitro and animal data, complete information regarding Chemistry, Manufacturing and Controls (CMC), and Clinical trial investigations in human participants. This characterization of the investigational product is optimized while being compliant with the regulations and GCPs.

Once all the necessary data to support a product's First-in-Human (FIH) study is available, the sponsor can prepare for the original or initial IND application submission.

The FDA's primary objectives in reviewing an IND are to assure the safety and rights of participants and to ensure the quality of the scientific evaluations of the molecule are adequate to permit an assessment of the drug's safety and effectiveness.

When a sponsor submits an IND, they are committing to certain obligations. Of key importance is ensuring trial participants' safety in the clinical conduct of the study, which is supported by science.

An IND is expected to be maintained and updated by the sponsor throughout the product's development lifecycle and reported on annually while in effect.

As per 21 CFR 312.22a

> *FDA's primary objectives in reviewing an IND are, in all phases of the investigation, to assure the safety and rights of subjects, and, in Phase 2 and 3, to help assure that the quality of the scientific evaluation of drugs is adequate to permit an evaluation*

of the drug's effectiveness and safety. Therefore, although FDA's review of Phase 1 submissions will focus on assessing the safety of Phase 1 investigations, FDA's review of Phases 2 and 3 submissions will also include an assessment of the scientific quality of the clinical investigations and the likelihood that the investigations will yield data capable of meeting statutory standards for marketing approval.

An IND is assembled in the Common Technical Document (CTD) format, which is the standard format for submitting applications, and other correspondence to CDER and CBER.

The CTD is the organization of information that is harmonized across various regions and presents "*all the Quality, Safety and Efficacy information in a common format*". This in turn has "*revolutionized the regulatory review processes enabling the implementation of good review practices*" globally. "*For industries, it has eliminated the need to reformat the information for submission to the different ICH regulatory authorities*".

The CTD is organized into five modules. Module 1 is region-specific and also contains administrative information specific to the sponsor; Modules 2, 3, 4, and 5 are intended to be common for all regions (Figure 1.2).

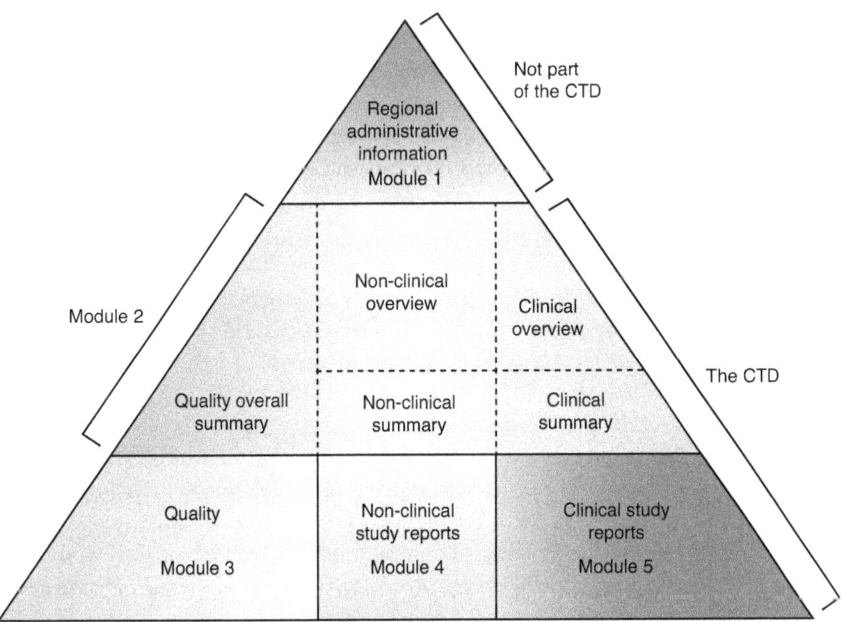

The CTD triangle. The Common Technical Document is organized into five modules. Module 1 is region specific and modules 2, 3, 4 and 5 are intended to be common for all regions.

FIGURE 1.2 The CTD. (https://www.ich.org/page/ctd.)

Contents of an IND (21 CFR 312.23)

Sec. 312.23 IND content and format.

a. *A sponsor who intends to conduct a clinical investigation subject to this part shall submit an "Investigational New Drug Application" (IND), including, in the following order:*
    1. *Cover sheet (Form FDA-1571). A cover sheet for the application contains the following:*
        i. *The name, address, and telephone number of the sponsor, the date of the application, and the name of the investigational new drug.*
        ii. *Identification of the phase or phases of the clinical investigation to be conducted.*
        iii. *A commitment not to begin clinical investigations until an IND covering the investigations is in effect.*
        iv. *A commitment that an Institutional Review Board (IRB) that complies with the requirements set forth in part 56 will be responsible for the initial and continuing review and approval of each of the studies in the proposed clinical investigation and that the investigator will report to the IRB proposed changes in the research activity in accordance with the requirements of part 56.*
        v. *A commitment to conduct the investigation in accordance with all other applicable regulatory requirements.*
        vi. *The name and title of the person responsible for monitoring the conduct and progress of the clinical investigations.*
        vii. *The name(s) and title(s) of the person(s) responsible under § 312.32 for the review and evaluation of information relevant to the safety of the drug.*
        viii. *If a sponsor has transferred any obligations for the conduct of any clinical study to a contract research organization, a statement containing the name and address of the contract research organization, identification of the clinical study, and a listing of the obligations transferred. If all obligations governing the conduct of the study have been transferred, a general statement of this transfer – in lieu of a listing of the specific obligations transferred – may be submitted.*
        ix. *The signature of the sponsor or the sponsor's authorized representative. If the person signing the application does not reside or have a place of business within the United States, the IND is required to contain the name and address of, and be countersigned by, an attorney, agent, or other authorized official who resides or maintains a place of business within the United States.*

As defined within 21 CFR 312.23 "Contents of an IND" an IND contains the following information:

Table of Contents – A list of all components of the IND. If submitted within the electronic Common Technical Document (eCTD) format (required of all commercial INDs), then the ToC is inherent within the eCTD backbone of the submission [11].

Core Information found within Module 1:

FDA Form 1571 (Cover Sheet) – Form 1571 provides the administrative information related to the sponsor (name, address, phone, and signature), name of the investigational product, date on which IND is submitted, phase of development being initiated, commitment to wait until IND is "effective", commitment to obtain Informed Consent and Institutional Review Board (IRB) review, trial monitoring identification, identification of the person responsible for safety evaluation and review of the product, and any sponsor obligations transferred to a Clinical Research Organization (CRO) or appropriate third-party.

Investigator's Brochure (IB) – The IB contains the complete information pertaining to the investigational product of what is known at the time of submission, including Chemistry, Manufacturing, and Controls, in vitro and in vivo data, pharmacokinetic data, animal data/toxicity studies, and past human experience (if available). The IB is expected to be reviewed by the sponsor annually (at a minimum) and updated with information throughout the product's development. New risks are added as they are identified, and the IB should be viewed by the sponsor as a living document that evolves as the development program progresses.

312.23 A(5) Investigator's brochure. If required under § 312.55, a copy of the investigator's brochure, containing the following information:

i. *A brief description of the drug substance and the formulation, including the structural formula, if known.*
ii. *A summary of the pharmacokinetics and biological disposition of the drug in animals and, if known, in humans.*

General Investigational Plan – plan for investigating the product for the following year, including the "kinds of clinical trials to be conducted in the first year following the submission (if plans are not developed for the entire year, the sponsor should so indicate); the estimated number of patients to be given the drug in those studies; and any risks of particular severity or seriousness anticipated on the basis of the toxicological data in animals or prior studies in humans with the drug or related drugs".

Core Information described within Module 2:

Summary Information – written and tabulated (where applicable) summaries for each key area of the product's characterization, formed from the basis of comprehensive information within the reports and data contained in the following modules related to Chemistry, Manufacturing, and Controls (CMC), Pharmacology and Toxicology, and Clinical.

Core Chemistry Manufacturing and Controls (CMC) information described within Module 3:

CMC Information – a section describing the composition, manufacture, and control of the drug substance (active pharmaceutical ingredient) and the drug product (active pharmaceutical ingredient plus excipients, fillers, etc.). CMC information also includes the methods, analytical procedures, and acceptable limits used "*to assure the identity, strength, quality, and purity of the drug product; and information sufficient to assure the product's stability during the planned clinical studies*". 21 CFR 312.23 (7)(iv)(a)(b).

A description of the product investigational labeling and an environmental risk assessment of the product fall within the CMC category; however, their corresponding information is typically placed within module 1.

Core Pharmacology and Toxicology information described within Module 4:

Pharmacology and Toxicology – pharmacological and toxicological data generated in vitro and in animals to ensure the proposed trials are adequately supported by nonclinical information (21 CFR 312.23). *(ii) A summary of the pharmacological and toxicological effects of the drug in animals and, to the extent known, in humans*

The kind, duration, and scope of animal and other tests required vary with the duration and nature of the proposed clinical trial investigation(s).

Core clinical information described within Module 5:

Clinical Trial Protocol and Related Information – the clinical trial protocol details the plan for the investigation and how the trial will be conducted. Additional information regarding the investigator(s) conducting the trial and their qualifications and agreement to IND regulations is also provided within this section of the application. Before any trial can commence at a specific investigator site, the IND safe-to-proceed is required from the FDA, and the Investigational Review Board (IRB) approval is also needed. Requirements and details regarding IRBs can be found in 21 CFR 56 and described further in Chapter 8.

IND Review Process

This chapter section describes the typical IND review process by the FDA, and what the sponsor can reasonably expect during this period.

Once a sponsor submits an IND, the FDA, as per CFR 312.20, will review the contents within 30 days of submission. The submission triggers a number of administrative procedures at the FDA's end, including the assignment of a Regulatory Health Project Manager (RPM), who becomes the sponsor's main point of contact. The RPM liaises within the respective FDA Division and obtains the FDA SME(s) reviewers within Medical, Toxicology, CMC, Clinical Pharmacology, Safety, and often Statistics. Depending on the nature of the molecule and the investigations planned, additional functional area reviewers could be assigned within FDA.

Usually, the FDA initial review determines if the application is complete in order to permit a substantive review. Any administrative or technical questions surrounding the application (if present) are quickly identified and raised with the sponsor, who can then address them.

Comments and potential deficiencies are then issued by the various FDA reviewers described above and provided to the sponsor via secure communications and correspondence from the FDA Project Manager.

The sponsor has the opportunity to address these comments and deficiencies in a timely manner during the 30-day review period, as agreed/requested by the FDA.

If deficiencies are adequately addressed by the sponsor within the 30-day review period, the FDA will issue a safe-to-proceed letter permitting shipment of the investigational product and initiation of the clinical trial described in the IND application, pending any agreements/changes made between the FDA and the sponsor during the review period. The IND is considered effective, and all IND requirements as per the CFR need to be adhered to (sections 21 CFR 312.30-33). Please also refer to the section related to IND maintenance in this chapter for additional information.

In some instances, the FDA may not issue a safe-to-proceed letter if no concerns are raised by the FDA during the IND review. No formal communication is required to activate an IND, but the sponsor must wait the required 30-day period before initiating the clinical trial.

If deficiencies are not sufficiently addressed within the 30-day period as determined by FDA review, a clinical hold is issued to the sponsor, meaning the sponsor cannot initiate their clinical investigation/trial until the hold is adequately addressed via a formal process (21 CFR 312.42).

Clinical studies conducted under 21 CFR 312 must be reviewed and approved by an Investigational Review Board (IRB) to safeguard the rights and welfare of human trial participants, confirm the scientific basis for the clinical research, and confirm the ethical considerations of the clinical research proposal.

IRBs and corresponding regulations will be discussed in further detail in subsequent chapters.

An Ethics Committee (EC) is the equivalent corresponding regulatory body governing, reviewing, and approving the same principles as an IRB in Europe and additional regions outside of the United States.

Clinical studies remain under periodic review by the IRB/EC, including all amendments and changes, and it is also the responsibility of the IRB/EC to ensure that the informed consent process is in place for the clinical study being reviewed.

IND Maintenance

An IND should be "maintained "throughout the product's development lifecycle, meaning all reporting requirements are adhered to and any new data on the molecule should be provided to the IND to enable the continual safety assessment of potential risks to human participants. New data supporting the various stages of the product should be submitted at the relevant time (for example, data to support a Phase 2 clinical trial design).

Protocol and Information Amendments

A sponsor can provide this information through different IND submission mechanisms, including Information Amendments (21 CFR 312.31), which allow for new animal data, changes, or updates to CMC or clinical information. Protocol amendments (21 CFR 312.30) are usually categorized as follows:

New Protocol – A sponsor can submit new protocols to an "open IND" if they are generally related to the molecule or within the same indication.

Change in Protocol – Ongoing clinical trials may be revised during their conduct for a number of reasons that commonly include a general change in design, a change in drug doses being evaluated, safety-related changes, and the addition of testing procedures to ensure participant safety. Changes to protocols should include a description of the change; it is a standard practice for the sponsor to submit a redlined and clean version of the protocol, replacing the original or prior version within the IND.

New Investigator – Sponsors shall inform the agency within 30 days of new investigators being added to the IND.

Safety Reports

21CFR312.32(c)(1)

IND safety reports. The sponsor must notify the FDA and all participating investigators (i.e., all investigators to whom the sponsor is providing drug under its INDs or under any investigator's IND) in an IND safety report of potential serious risks from clinical trials or any other source, as soon as possible, but in no case later than 15 calendar days after the sponsor determines that the information qualifies for reporting under paragraphs (c)(1)(i), (c)(1)(ii), (c)(1)(iii), or (c)(1)(iv) of this section. In each IND safety report, the sponsor must identify all IND safety reports previously submitted to the FDA concerning a similar suspected adverse reaction and must analyze the significance of the suspected adverse reaction in light of previous, similar reports or any other relevant information.

21 CFR 312.32 states that the sponsor will notify the FDA and all participating investigators in an IND Safety Report no later than 15 calendar days after the sponsor receives the information if:

- Any adverse experience associated with the use of the drug is **Serious** and **Unexpected**.

- Any finding from tests in laboratory animals suggests a significant risk to humans participating in the investigational trials involving the product.

Typically, once the safety event information is provided to the sponsor, a designated team meets to assess the event and potential causality and relatedness, etc., and determines the reporting criteria for the FDA. The assessment is done in a timely manner, and each sponsor adheres to well-documented internal procedures for triggering the starting clock for the calendar day reporting timeline. There are additional aspects of safety reporting that are not covered in this chapter but that can be found in detail within 21 CFR 312.32.

Annual Reports

A sponsor shall, within 60 days of the anniversary date that the IND went into effect, submit a brief report of the progress of the investigation that includes:

> a. *Individual study information. A brief summary of the status of each study in progress and each study completed during the previous year. The summary is required to include the following information for each study:*

In accordance with 21 CFR 312.33, the sponsor is required to submit an annual report within 60 days of the anniversary date that IND became effective. Aspects of what is expected to be provided to the FDA are described in the CFR. It is worth noting that in 2011, the FDA adopted the ICH's 2010 guidance, "The Development Safety Update Report, E2F", and began accepting the Development Safety Update Report (DSUR) in place of the IND annual report, with the caveat that all aspects of 21 CFR 312.33 are accounted for in the DSUR. Since the DSUR is accepted globally, this has enabled sponsor's to streamline their annual reporting procedures to regulatory authorities for investigational products, with regional appendices to the Global DSUR capturing specific information as needed [12].

NDA PROCESS AND LIFECYCLE MANAGEMENT

Through the data collected via the IND process and similar global mechanisms (for example, Clinical Trial Applications) throughout the product's lifecycle, sufficient evidence may be obtained to form the basis of registration or application for the new drug. When a sponsor determines that the data generated supports the safe and effective use of the product in the studied patient population, the sponsor must then submit for FDA review this information in the form of an NDA to demonstrate that this safety and efficacy have met all requirements as per regulations. If the investigational product is a biological or vaccine, the equivalent application is referred to as a Biologics License Application (BLA). Globally, this is referred to as a marketing authorization application (MAA).

What is an NDA?

The New Drug Application is a package of required data and reports regarding the product's manufacturing process, animal studies and clinical trial evaluations that should in total demonstrate that the drug is safe and effective in its proposed use and that the benefits of the drug outweigh the risks for patients in the treatment setting or indication. In general, the NDA package provides the results of all pertinent evaluations conducted under the respective product's IND, including the aforementioned information and information regarding how the drug behaves in the body and how it is manufactured, processed, and packaged so that it demonstrates these aspects are adequate to preserve its identity, purity, strength, and quality.

Before submitting the NDA, a sponsor typically engages in dialogue with the FDA review team assigned to their product in a pre-NDA meeting, which is usually solicited at the time of pivotal trial data results, which will form the basis for registration. Key agreements with the agency can be obtained via this important meeting, and this also provides the sponsor with an opportunity to address any potential questions or concerns from the agency raised in this meeting, in advance of the NDA submission.

Contents of an NDA 21 CFR 314

Like the IND application, the CTD format also forms the basis of the NDA, though different information is usually required to support registration. The CTD modules are the same as described in the section on INDs.

Briefly, as per 21 CFR 314.50, the key components of the NDA are as follows:

FDA Form 356H – name and address of the sponsor, date of submission, category of submission, name of product (including research codes, INN, and proposed brand or trade name), all referenced INDs for the product, and the proposed indication for use.

The 356H form also captures whether this product is intended as a prescription and allows for the sponsor to check which aspects of the application are included in the filing package.

Labeling (US Prescribing Information) – a guide to physicians and prescribers on how to use the drug for their patients, with the information providing an overview of the benefits and risks. The proposed labeling text included in the NDA is a condensed set of scientific highlights "*with annotations to the information in the summary and technical sections of the NDA that support the inclusion of each statement in the labeling*". Please refer to 21 CFR 314.50(c).2(i) and also the FDA website regarding Prescribing Information Resources for more information [13].

Module 2 summaries include:

- CMC information for the proposed marketed product.
- Nonclinical pharmacology and toxicology
- Human pharmacokinetics and bioavailability.
- Microbiology (for anti-infective drugs only).

- Clinical data, including the results of statistical analyses of the clinical trials.
- The sponsor should also provide information that presents the benefits and risk considerations related to the drug, including a discussion of any proposed additional studies or surveillance the applicant intends to conduct post-marketing.

These summaries are created from the data and reports located in the corresponding sections of the NDA within Modules 3, 4, and 5, which are usually referred to as the technical sections of the NDA.

Module 3 (CMC) contains all CMC-related information pertaining to the product's drug substance and drug product manufacturing processes, methods, and controls. It describes the intended commercial dosage form and formulation for proposed patient use and should contain sufficient information regarding the development of the drug product, including excipient and container-closure information.

Module 4 Nonclinical contains all study reports of nonclinical testing and evaluations of the drug, from its initial development during the IND stage through the NDA. There should be sufficient nonclinical data at the time of the NDA filing to support the proposed use in the intended patient population and corresponding product labeling.

Module 5 Clinical contains all reports and data of all pertinent clinical study information to support the drug's proposed use in the intended patient population. This section of the NDA should also provide for the integrated Summaries of Clinical Safety and Clinical Efficacy, often referred to as ISS and ISE, respectively. Module 5 is often viewed as the key section of the NDA, as this is where the FDA's review team focuses on the safety and efficacy of the product in the patient population for intended use, based on the clinical trials completed over the course of the product lifecycle to that point.

In addition to the information described within each module, additional areas of a sponsor's NDA contain patent certifications, Bioresearch Monitoring, Case Report Tabulations, and datasets in various FDA-required formats (SDTM, SEND, ADaM, etc.).

Depending on the clinical trial data supporting the proposed indication, a product may be required to have a Risk Evaluation and Mitigation Strategy (REMS) to ensure its safe use in the patient population. A REMS may have various components and can include a simple communication plan or "elements to assure safe use", which may involve prescriber training and certification. For additional information on REMS, refer to Ref. [14].

Overall, the FDA's cross-disciplinary review team, comprised of experts in their respective fields, reviews each aspect of the NDA and provides a conclusion for that area, which is then pulled together in the form of an overall benefit-risk determination of the product. The FDA also audits the sponsor and certain clinical trial sites to ensure the quality of the clinical trial and corresponding data.

NDA Review Process

The FDA reviews the NDA submission on a timeline typically defined by two categories [15]:

Standard (S): The total timeline typically takes 12 months (2 months for determining whether the application is fileable and 10 months for review).
Priority (P): The total timeline typically takes 8 months (2 months for determining whether the application is fileable and 8 months for review).

In certain cases, approval of the new drug can occur much sooner than these designated timelines, especially in instances of oncology products or products intended to treat rare and serious diseases where patients have limited treatment options. In these cases, expedited timelines can be employed by the FDA review team, with the determination of an approval issued well in advance of the PDUFA goal date.

In general, there are well-defined stages of the NDA review process, which include various communications and opportunities to discuss the application with the FDA.

These communications include:

Day 74 (S)/Day 60(P) Filing Letter, where the FDA has reached a determination that the NDA can be filed (is considered complete to permit a substantive review). The action date is cited in this letter to the sponsor.
Information Requests (IRs) issued by the FDA reviewers across multi-disciplinary areas occur on a rolling basis throughout the NDA review cycle. Often, initial IRs focus on the content of the application and where certain information is located within the eCTD. Once the substantive review is initiated by the FDA reviewers, the IRs become more content-oriented, with questions spanning across each module, corresponding to CMC information, statistical analyses, safety information, clinical trial data, and clinical pharmacology analyses.
Mid-Cycle Communication often occurs as a teleconference with the FDA review team, in which the sponsor is informed of any potential deficiencies in the application or areas for clarification or follow-up. This communication is also issued in the form of a formal letter from the FDA to the sponsor.
Late-Cycle Communication, much like mid-cycle communication, usually takes place as a teleconference with the FDA, corresponding to a formal letter/ minutes. Any potential post-marketing requirements or commitments are highlighted at this stage in the NDA, as are potential labeling timelines, if these haven't been discussed prior between the FDA and the sponsor.
Action (Decision) Letter is the formal communication to the sponsor once the FDA has reached a decision on the approvability of the NDA. Action letters typically fall into either "approval" or "complete responses". A "Complete Response" letter details the actions a sponsor needs to undertake to address the deficiencies. The FDA review team determined the NDA was not approvable in its current form.

NDA Maintenance

Conceptually very similar to IND maintenance, NDA/BLA maintenance is the responsibility of the sponsor and must be conducted in accordance with local regulations and guidelines.

All new labeling and substantial CMC amendments must be submitted and approved by the FDA before implementation.

The sponsor must continue to collect, analyze, and review safety data in the post-approval setting and abide by safety-reporting regulations [16].

A periodic safety update report, typically referred to in the US as the Periodic Adverse Drug Event Report (PADER), but also referred to as per ICH terminology as the Periodic Benefit-Risk Evaluation Report (PBRER), is used to satisfy the periodic post-marketing safety reporting requirements in 21 CFR 314.80(c)(2) and 21 CFR 600.80(c).

These reports must be submitted quarterly to the NDA for the first 3 years following the approval date and annually thereafter. The periodic safety reports must contain specific information outlined in the regulations cited.

The NDA/BLA Annual Report must be submitted to the application each year within 60 days of the anniversary date of the drug's US approval. The annual report should contain information as required by 21 CFR 314.81(b)(2), including a summary of new research information related to the drug, labeling changes that occurred during the reporting year and distribution data for the FDA to review. A summary of new clinical safety and efficacy information, CMC information, and updates on the progress of any post-marketing requirements and commitments are also provided within this report.

HOW GCPs PLAY A ROLE IN THE IND/NDA SUBMISSION AND LIFECYCLE

It is well recognized that GCPs are essential to help ensure the safety of trial participants as well as the integrity of the data generated from trials. As such, it is key for all functional areas within a company to partner with Quality Assurance from the very beginning of initiating IND-enabling nonclinical studies and forming clinical development plans for efficacy. This is essential because all Good Laboratory Practices (GLPs), Good Manufacturing Practices (GMPs), and GCPs should be adhered to and considered throughout a product's life cycle. Data generated and collected by the sponsor during animal studies, manufacturing/pharmaceutical development, and human clinical trials conducted under an IND form the basis of the NDA/BLA.

Key areas of focus for GCPs are inherent within clinical trial conduct, the selection of qualified investigators to conduct the study, IRBs, data collection methods and integrity, and overall compliance: compliance with regulations and adherence to the clinical study protocol and any changes/amendments introduced during the study's lifecycle.

Any clinical trial protocol deviations should be documented accordingly, captured appropriately within the sponsor's record-keeping processes, and in accordance with GCPs.

Bioresearch monitoring is an area in which the FDA has the authority to inspect and audit research data and corresponding records. This monitoring spans across multiple areas of compliance responsibility, including the sponsor, the investigator, the IRB, and also nonclinical laboratory compliance.

As per the FDA's Bioresearch Monitoring Program Information,

> *the BIMO program was established to assure the quality and integrity of data submitted to the agency in support of new product approvals and marketing applications, as well as, to provide for protection of the rights and welfare of the thousands of human subjects and animals involved in FDA regulated research.* [17]

As can be seen, GCPs are interwoven in all aspects of drug development, and a sponsor that creates its working processes within this framework is ensuring success for the next steps in a product's lifecycle: when that product has demonstrated a clinical efficacy benefit for trial participants and is safe, then the NDA can be developed for submission to a regulatory body, such as the FDA, to approve its use for patients within the proposed indication.

REGULATORY FAQS

WHEN SHOULD WE START IND APPLICATION PLANNING?

A prudent timeline is typically 6–12 months before a sponsor targets for an IND submission, given that animal studies and CMC processes should have already been initiated and adequately characterized to support the submission.

HOW OFTEN DOES AN INVESTIGATOR'S BROCHURE (IB) HAVE TO BE UPDATED?

The expectation is for sponsors to review the IB at a minimum annually and assess the information to be updated. IBs should also be updated before the annual review timeline if new substantial safety or product information is obtained. Please refer to ICH E6 and 21 CFR 312.55 for more information.

DOES THE FDA PROVIDE COMMENTS ON EVERY PROTOCOL SUBMISSION WITHIN 30 DAYS?/IS THERE APPROVAL FOR EVERY PROTOCOL SUBMITTED TO THE FDA?

The short answer is no. Once an original IND is opened, new protocols can be submitted to the effective IND. The FDA reviews all protocols submitted but may or may not issue any comments on that specific protocol or protocol package. FDA typically doesn't issue official safe-to-proceeds for each new protocol (but may sometimes). It's important to note that there is no mandate in the CFR for a sponsor to "wait" the 30 days after submission of a new protocol to an open IND, nor is it mandated that the FDA be required to review the protocol within those 30 days if it is submitted to an active IND. However, it is good practice to wait for a period of time (many sponsors choose 30 days) while your GRA representative engages with their FDA RPM contact in the expectation of any forthcoming comments from the FDA Review Team. If FDA review of certain parts of the protocol is desired, then it is recommended that the cover letter of the protocol submission include this request.

WILL THE FDA ACCEPT EX-US DATA FROM TRIALS/SITES CONDUCTED OUTSIDE OF THE US TO SUPPORT AN NDA?

Yes. As per 21 CFR 312.120 and the 2012 FDA Guidance for Industry, ex-US data that is generated from studies conducted according to GCPs can be used to support NDAs, as most sponsor trials are conducted globally [18]. Usually, US trial sites are conducted under the IND, and all CFR requirements are expected to be met. Ex-US sites are not conducted under the IND and therefore not subject to the specificities per CFR, such as FDA Form 1572.

CAN WE INITIATE A TRIAL ONCE WE SUBMIT THE PROTOCOL TO THE FDA?

If the protocol is part of an original IND application, then the sponsor is required to either wait for the safe-to-proceed to be issued by the FDA or wait the required 30-day period. In addition, IRB approval is required for the trial site prior to the trial being initiated there.

If the IND is already "opened", then refer to the corresponding previous question. IRB approval must be obtained before initiating the trial at the clinical site.

ARE WE REQUIRED TO REGISTER OUR CLINICAL STUDY ON CLINTRIALS.GOV?

Not necessarily, as it depends on the clinical trial being conducted. A checklist is available to help sponsor's evaluate if the study is an Applicable Clinical Study (ACT), requiring registration on clintrials.gov [19].

It's worth noting that many sponsors choose the more conservative route of registering the study, if any gray area exists.

WHAT IF YOU DON'T HAVE AN NCT NUMBER YET FOR FORM 3674 SUBMISSION TO THE IND?

The recommended approach is to complete FDA Form 3674 and enter a placeholder (usually a string of zeroes) for the NCT number in the form (the current forms won't allow a sponsor to leave this section blank). The sponsor should also inform the agency in the cover letter that this trial meets the criteria of an applicable clinical study and will be registered on clinicaltrials.gov; however, the NCT number is not yet available. Then, once the NCT number is obtained, a new 3674 form can be submitted at the time of the next submission for that particular study, informing the agency that the trial was registered and the number was obtained.

DO SPONSOR TRANSFER OF OBLIGATION FORMS NEED TO BE SUBMITTED TO THE FDA?

Yes. It is expected that all sponsor obligations as per 21 CFR 312.52 be communicated in writing to the FDA. FDA Form 1571, which is part of an IND submission, has a specific place where the sponsor needs to acknowledge if any of the sponsor's obligations are transferred. Accordingly, a "Transfer of Obligations" document should be submitted with the form/IND submission. This Transfer of Sponsor Obligations should be updated accordingly throughout a product lifecyle per clinical study conducted under the IND.

WHAT DOES 30 DAYS MEAN WHEN WE ADD INVESTIGATORS TO A CLINICAL STUDY (RE THE 30-DAY TIMELINE TO SUBMIT THE INFORMATION TO THE FDA)?

Investigators should be added to the IND in a timely manner, which is specified in the CFR as within 30 days of being added to the clinical study. The sponsor should determine the 30-day trigger that starts the clock in a well-defined process that is adhered to for consistency. Day 0 to start the clock is often considered the day the investigator's site receives the clinical study drug shipment for the trial, or it can be the date when the investigator signs the FDA Form 1572 (Statement of Investigator). Often, the new investigators or investigator updates are batched within a 30-day period and submitted as one submission to the IND in a periodical manner.

WHAT INFORMATION IS NEEDED TO SUBMIT NEW PROTOCOL PACKAGES TO THE FDA, IF NOT A NEW IND?

The new protocol submission should be a package that adequately permits the FDA review of the protocol and the corresponding implementation of said trial conduct. Often, this package, in addition to the new protocol, may include the model ICFs, new investigator information, Transfer of Sponsor Obligations, and any corresponding CMC or nonclinical data to support the objective of the trial.

WHEN SHOULD NDA PLANNING START?

It's prudent for a sponsor to begin planning for the NDA 12–18 months in advance of a targeted submission. This allows for thorough preparation of submission documents, SMEs understanding the data in a cross-collaborative team setting, identifying and mitigating risks, and planning for health authority meetings and inspections.

IF THE STUDY IS CONDUCTED IN THE US-ONLY, SHOULD AN IND ANNUAL REPORT OR THE DEVELOPMENT SAFETY UPDATE REPORT (DSUR) BE SUBMITTED?

Though an IND Annual Report is required by regulations (21 CFR 312.33), the FDA has accepted the DSUR in lieu of the AR since approximately 2011, with the issuance of its DSUR Guidance [12]. As of this writing, the FDA has taken it one step further and proposed a regulation change in December 2022 for IND annual reporting, suggesting that acceptance of the DSUR instead of the IND AR would satisfy the CFR requirement.

WHAT IS THE EXPECTED TIMEFRAME FOR THE SUBMISSION OF A CSR AFTER THE STUDY IS COMPLETED?

In general, though a specific timeline is not mandated in the US CFR, in the EU it is expected that a clinical study report (or synopsis) will be available no later than 12 months from the last-patient-last-visit of the clinical trial. Sponsors aim to adhere to this timeframe when conducting multi-national global trials.

WHAT IS THE AVERAGE TIME FRAME FOR IND TO NDA APPROVAL?

It depends on the disease and the unmet needs for patients. Typical timelines for a product's development through NDA approval may span approximately 5–10 years and sometimes longer, but exceptions are made by regulators. GCP principles should be incorporated as early as possible in Phase 1 evaluations since the traditional paradigms are not always followed. For examples of expedited development timeline approvals, please refer to the original US NDA approvals of Zykadia® and Ibrance®, available at drugs@fda.gov:

https://www.accessdata.fda.gov/scripts/cder/daf/index.cfm

REFERENCES

[1] International Council for Harmonisation of Technical Requirements for Pharmaceuticals for Human Use (ICH) (November 2016). *Integrated Addendum to ICH E6 (R1): Guideline for Good Clinical Practice E6 (R2).*

[2] US Food and Drug Administration Regulations: *Good Clinical Practice and Clinical Trials.* https://www.fda.gov/science-research/clinical-trials-and-human-subject-protection/regulations-good-clinical-practice-and-clinical-trials

[3] US Food and Drug Administration. https://www.fda.gov/

[4] US Food and Drug Administration. Organization. https://www.fda.gov/about-fda/fda-organization/fda-organization-charts

[5] US Food and Drug Administration. *Federal Food, Drug, and Cosmetic Act (FD&C Act).*

[6] US Food and Drug Administration. *Part II: 1938, Food, Drug, Cosmetic Act.* https://www.fda.gov/about-fda/changes-science-law-and-regulatory-authorities/part-ii-1938-food-drug-cosmetic-act#:~:text=FDR%20signed%20the%20Food%2C%20Drug, adequate%20directions%20for%20safe%20use.

[7] Office of the Federal Registrar. Code of Federal Regulations. https://www.archives.gov/federal-register/cfr#:~:text=The%20Code%20of%20Federal%20Regulations%20(CFR)%20presents%20the%20official%20and,fashion%20in%20a%20single%20publication.&text=The%20CFR%20is%20updated%20by,version%20of%20any%20given%20rule

[8] U.S. Department of Health and Human Services. Food and Drug Administration. Center for Drug Evaluation and Research (CDER). Center for Biologics Evaluation and Research (CBER) (September 2023). *Formal Meetings between the FDA and Sponsors or Applicants of PDUFA Products. Draft Guidance for Industry.* https://www.fda.gov/regulatory-information/search-fda-guidance-documents/formal-meetings-between-fda-and-sponsors-or-applicants-pdufa-products

[9] European Medicines Agency. *Scientific Advice and Protocol Assistance.* https://www.ema.europa.eu/en/human-regulatory-overview/research-and-development/scientific-advice-and-protocol-assistance#:~:text=EMA%20gives%20scientific%20advice%20by,advice%20on%20the%20developer's%20proposals

[10] US Food and Drug Administration. *Investigational New Drug (IND) Application.* https://www.fda.gov/drugs/types-applications/investigational-new-drug-ind-application

[11] US Food and Drug Administration. *Electronic Common Technical Document (eCTD).* https://www.fda.gov/drugs/electronic-regulatory-submission-and-review/electronic-common-technical-document-ectd

[12] U.S. Department of Health and Human Services. Food and Drug Administration. Center for Drug Evaluation and Research (CDER). Center for Biologics Evaluation and Research (CBER) (August 2011). *E2F Development Safety Update Report Guidance for Industry.* https://www.fda.gov/files/drugs/published/E2F-Development-Safety-Update-Report.pdf

[13] US Food and Drug Administration (n.d.). *Prescribing Information Resources.* https://www.fda.gov/drugs/fdas-labeling-resources-human-prescription-drugs/prescribing-information-resources

[14] U.S. Department of Health and Human Services. Food and Drug Administration. Center for Drug Evaluation and Research (CDER). Center for Biologics Evaluation and Research (CBER) (January 2023). *Format and Content of a REMS Document. Guidance for Industry.* https://www.fda.gov/media/77846/download

[15] US Food and Drug Administration (n.d.). *CDER 21st Century Review Process Desk Reference Guide.* https://www.fda.gov/media/78941/download

[16] U.S. Department of Health and Human Services. Food and Drug Administration. Center for Drug Evaluation and Research (CDER). Center for Biologics Evaluation and Research (CBER) (March 2001). *Postmarketing Safety Reporting for Human Drug and Biological Products Including Vaccines. Guidance for Industry.* https://www.fda.gov/media/73593/download

[17] US Food and Drug Administration. *Bioresearch Monitoring Program Information.* https://www.fda.gov/inspections-compliance-enforcement-and-criminal-investigations/fda-bioresearch-monitoring-information/bioresearch-monitoring-program-information

[18] U.S. Department of Health and Human Services. Food and Drug Administration. Center for Drug Evaluation and Research (CDER). Center for Biologics Evaluation and Research (CBER) (March 2012). *FDA Acceptance of Foreign Clinical Studies Not Conducted Under an IND Frequently Asked Questions. Guidance for Industry.* https://www.fda.gov/media/83209/download

[19] National Institutes of Health. Clinical trials.gov, Applicable Study Checklist. https://prsinfo.clinicaltrials.gov/ACT_Checklist.pdf

2 Principles of Good Clinical Practice (GCP)

John S. Klein and Sonya T. Edgerton

BRIEF HISTORY OF ICH AND GCP

As early as the 1960s and 1970s, product registration controls began to emerge across many countries, often driven by prior tragedies, the most famous being the Thalidomide scandal,[1] which were linked to poorly controlled pharmaceutical development. This period saw an increase in formalized laws, regulations, and guidelines that would focus on the evaluation of data on the safety, quality, and efficacy of new products. The outcome, however, resulted in duplicating efforts, increased costs, and extended product development timelines necessary to gain approval for new products around the globe. The movement toward a harmonized approach began to grow in the 1980s, when Europe started to establish a single market for product development. The stakeholders in the development of a harmonized approach were expanded to include the United States and Japan when it was recognized that streamlining efforts across these regions would improve the medical product development process.

These realities spawned the formation of the International Council of Harmonisation (ICH) in 1990. The initial work of ICH focused on harmonizing the standards of safety, quality, and efficacy as the basis for approving and authorizing new medicinal products. Over time, harmonization efforts have grown and expanded to other global regions and have become the global standard for drug and device development.

ICH guidelines continue to evolve and grow. The current guidelines are widely used throughout the industry, and revisions continue to further focus on the safety, rights, and well-being of patients while improving quality by providing a globally standardized approach. We will focus on one specific section of these guidelines – E6 – Good Clinical Practice (GCP), first released in 1996. This section is within the Efficacy Guideline category, which focuses on the design, conduct, safety, and reporting of clinical trials, novel types of medicines, and techniques to produce targeted medicines.

ICH E6 – GOOD CLINICAL PRACTICE

"Good Clinical Practice is an international ethical and scientific quality standard for designing, conducting, recording, and reporting trials that involve the participation of human subjects."[2] The initial guideline described the responsibilities and

DOI: 10.1201/9781003407010-2

expectations for the conduct of clinical trials. It covers all participants, including investigators, monitors, sponsors, and Institutional Review Boards (IRB), and addresses activities such as monitoring trial data, reporting, and archiving clinical trials, Essential Documents, as well as the Investigator's Brochure.

Over time, this guideline has been amended to expand its focus on ensuring human subject protection and the reliability of trial results. These changes further encourage the implementation of improved and efficient approaches to trial design, conduct, oversight, recording, and reporting. As clinical trials expand in scale, complexity, and cost, GCP has been expanded to include the growing use of technology in clinical trials as well as increasing the application of risk management processes to further the focus on efficiency and quality.

GCP has become an international standard for how to conduct clinical trials. It provides the basis for how investigators, monitors, and sponsors work to ensure clinical trials protect the safety and rights of subjects while generating quality trial results. The guidelines provide a framework for how research is to be conducted without being overly proscriptive. In this way, GCP guidelines form the foundation, or starting point, of how clinical trial work is to be conducted. It is up to sponsors, monitors, and investigators to define how they will implement these guidelines to optimize quality, reduce risk, and protect subjects. This is ultimately how they will be evaluated by regulatory agencies through inspections and audits.

The ICH E6(R2) GCP guideline is structured concisely[3,4]:

- Glossary
- The Principles of ICH GCP
- Institutional Review Board/Independent Ethics Committee (IRB/IEC)
- Investigator
- Sponsor
- Clinical Trial Protocol and Protocol Amendments
- Investigator's Brochure
- Essential Documents

Each of these sections provides guidance on what is expected, but the 'how' it is to be done is left to the sponsor, monitor, or investigator. A closer look at each of these sections is warranted.

GLOSSARY

The glossary section provides standardized definitions for the key terms used throughout the GCP guideline. These definitions give users a common understanding of key industry terms and acronyms.

> **Implementation Tip** – As sponsors, monitors, and investigators build written procedures, refer to and use these as standard definitions wherever possible. Customized definitions that build on these standards also work, but be sure to use them as the starting point to help build a culture of compliance and general common understanding.

THE PRINCIPLES OF GCP

The first of the principles sets the tone for the overall intent of GCP: "Clinical trials should be conducted in accordance with the ethical principles that have their origin in the Declaration of Helsinki and that are consistent with GCP and the applicable regulatory requirement(s)."[5] Ethical considerations must always be at the forefront of trial design and conduct, as well as subject safety and privacy.

These general principles are woven throughout the fabric of GCP. Some of the key concepts they touch on include:

- Identifying and weighing foreseeable risks against trial benefits;
- Placing the rights, safety, and well-being of trial subjects as an over-riding consideration;
- Ensuring nonclinical and clinical data on the investigational product adequately support the clinical trial design;
- Ensuring the scientific soundness of the clinical trial design;
- Conducting trial activities following an Institutional Review Board/Independent Ethics Committee (IRB/IEC)-approved protocol;
- Providing medical care using qualified physicians/dentists, and confirming that everyone involved in the trial has appropriate training and qualifications;
- Obtaining voluntary informed consent from research participants prior to initiating trial activities;
- Recording clinical trial information/data accurately and maintaining confidentiality;
- Manufacturing investigational products following Good Manufacturing Practice (GMP);
- Implementing systems that ensure quality in all aspects of a trial to facilitate human subject protection and the reliability of trial results.

Subsequent chapters in this book will outline expectations for these key principles and how best to implement them.

INSTITUTIONAL REVIEW BOARD/INDEPENDENT ETHICS COMMITTEE (IRB/IEC)

The IRB/IEC has a pivotal role in safeguarding the rights, safety, and well-being of clinical trial subjects. These boards/committees act as gatekeepers and provide oversight to ensure the clinical trial is sound, and subjects under their purview are taken care of through qualified medical providers and consent freely to participation in the trial.

IRB/IEC members must review trial documents, including the clinical trial protocol and any amendments, the Investigator's Brochure, a written consent form (original and institutionally modified), any compensation that may be provided to trial subjects, and other relevant written documentation. The IRB/IEC must also provide a written review of the documents provided and their recommendation on whether to approve or not approve trial conduct.

A more detailed look at the responsibilities, composition, procedures, and record requirements of the IRB/IEC can be found in Chapter 8.

Implementation Tip – Institutions and stand-alone IRB/IEC should have written procedures for the formation, qualifications, and conduct of these committees. The procedures should reflect the requirements of GCP and governing regulatory authorities and be available for review by auditors and inspectors as needed.

INVESTIGATOR

Investigator's Qualifications and Agreements

The investigator plays a pivotal role in GCP and clinical trial conduct by facilitating informed consent, providing medical care, providing safety oversight, and documenting clinical trial data. Each investigator should be qualified (education, training, and experience) to properly conduct the clinical trial. Each investigator will be required to provide a curriculum vita to the sponsor and regulatory authorities to demonstrate their qualifications. In addition, the investigator and their staff should work in compliance with GCP and other regulatory requirements.

Implementation Tip – Each investigator and all personnel at the site/institution who are working on the clinical trial site should be trained in the principles of GCP as well as any procedures the site/institution has pertaining to clinical research. These training records and procedures should be available for review at a pre-study visit or site initiation visit, as well as during a site audit or inspection by regulatory authorities.

Throughout a trial, each investigator must provide access for monitors and the sponsor to inspect and audit clinical trial source data, facilities, protocol compliance, training, and adequate record-keeping. In addition, the investigator has a responsibility for overseeing any personnel who perform activities on behalf of the investigator at the clinical trial location.

Medical Care of Trial Subjects

The investigator is responsible for all trial-related medical (or dental) decisions and must be a qualified physician (or dentist). Investigators ensure that adequate medical care is provided to all trial subjects, including any care required for adverse events related to the trial. In addition, the investigator has a responsibility to view the subject holistically and notify their primary care physician about participation in the trial, where appropriate.

Communication with IRB/IEC

Investigators have a responsibility for communicating with the IRB/IEC for all trial-related concerns, including submission of the protocol, informed consent, and other written information. As documents are updated throughout the trial, updates and amendments should also be submitted for IRB/IEC review. As the investigator receives communications and approvals/favorable opinions/withdrawals of approval from the IRB/IEC, these should be shared with the sponsor. The sponsor should have a process for liaising with the IRB/IEC throughout a trial to ensure continuity of communication between the sponsor, investigator, and IRB/IEC.

Compliance with Protocol

A key responsibility for the investigator is to conduct the trial in compliance with the protocol as approved by regulatory authorities and the IRB/IEC. It is also necessary for the investigator to sign the protocol or contract to confirm their agreement to conduct the trial. When deviations from the protocol occur, the investigator should document these deviations as required by the protocol and notify the IRB/IEC and sponsor.

Implementation Tip – The importance of protocol compliance cannot be understated. In addition to signing the protocol and contract, the investigator has an obligation to keep the safety and rights of trial subjects at the forefront of their work. Investigative sites should have processes in place to show compliance with GCP as well as local regulations. CFR312.60 specifically highlights the responsibilities of the investigator in this regard, and directed regulatory actions have been taken against investigators/sites that do not uphold these requirements.

Investigational Product(s)

The investigator maintains responsibility for the investigational product for the trial site. While some of these responsibilities may be shared with a pharmacist or other appropriate individual, the accountability for investigational material remains with the investigator. Accurate records of investigational material at the trial site are required to ensure accurate randomization and blinding (as appropriate), as well as the final disposition of all investigational material at the end of the trial.

Informed Consent of Trial Subjects

One of the most important responsibilities an investigator has is to obtain informed consent for each subject. There are several requirements for the content of an informed consent document, how consent is to be obtained, and the rights a subject has before, during, and after participation in a trial. A more in-depth look at the informed consent requirements and processes can be found in Chapter 6.

Records and Reports

Investigators and site personnel must maintain accurate source documentation and trial records at all times that reflect the observations and treatment of each subject. All data is expected to maintain ALCOA-C standards (attributable, legible, contemporaneous, original, accurate, and complete), and changes should be traceable and documented. Timely data capture is important to ensure adequate monitoring and reporting by the sponsor. In addition to record keeping during a trial, there are expectations that trial documents are maintained at the site as specified in Essential Documents for the Conduct of a Clinical Trial (see below) and as required by local regulatory authorities. These documents should be retained until at least 2 years after the last approval of a marketing application in an ICH region or longer as specified by regulation. The sponsor has a responsibility to notify the investigator when documents are no longer needed to be retained.

The financial aspects of the trial, and any other financial interests the investigator may have, should be documented in a formal agreement. A more detailed discussion of financial disclosure requirements can be found in Chapter 7.

Progress Reports

As the trial progresses, the investigator should submit written progress summaries of the trial status to the IRB/IEC at least annually, or as requested, and should also notify the sponsor and IRB/IEC of any changes that occur that may impact the conduct of the trial and/or subject safety.

Safety Reporting

The investigator has a responsibility to report safety issues that occur during the conduct of a trial. All serious adverse events (SAEs) should be reported to the sponsor immediately unless otherwise specified, and if additional information is requested, it should be provided in a timely manner. Further detail on clinical trial safety reporting is covered in Chapter 5.

Premature Termination Or Suspension of a Trial

Even if a trial is suspended or prematurely terminated for any reason, it is the responsibility of the investigator to inform the trial participants and provide any follow-up and treatments as required. GCP provides guidance on several scenarios of trial suspension or early termination and what is to be done and who should be notified, including any follow-up therapies that should be provided to the trial subjects.

Final Report(s) by the Investigator

Once the trial is complete, the investigator should notify the IRB/IEC and provide them with a summary of the trial outcomes (clinical study report) when available.

SPONSOR

A sponsor of a clinical trial is required to put in place a system to manage quality throughout all stages of the clinical trial process. Quality should include the overall protection of human subjects as well as ensuring efficient trial design and conduct that focus on the reliability of the trial.

Quality Management

To adequately include quality in clinical trials, the sponsor should assess the risks that are inherent in a trial and balance these against the quality measures being implemented. One component of this is to ensure all parts of the trial are operationally feasible and avoid unnecessary complexity, procedures, and data collection efforts. All components of the trial, from protocols to case report forms and other documents, should be clear, concise, and consistent to ensure quality and reduce risk. To manage overall risk, sponsors should implement a quality management system that utilizes a risk-based approach that includes[6]:

- Critical Processes and Data Identification
- Risk Identification
- Risk Evaluation
- Risk Control
- Risk Communication
- Risk Review
- Risk Reporting

To manage risk and best support quality, a sponsor should implement and maintain quality assurance and quality control systems with written SOPs. This will ensure trials are conducted in their entirety (including data generated and reported) in compliance with GCP and regulatory requirements. In addition, the sponsor is responsible for ensuring access to all clinical trial documents and data, including those at a trial site, for audits and inspections.

Implementation Tip – Sponsors should implement a quality management system that includes overall quality policies and processes. These should include, but not be limited to, a Quality Policy; Procedural Document Management; Good Documentation Practices & Data Integrity; Training Management; Vendor Selection, Qualification, and Oversight; and Management Review; and Managing Deviations, Escalations, and Corrective & Preventive Actions.

Implementation Tip – Conducting trial feasibility to assess the logistics of conducting the trial across the countries/regions being considered is an important step in trial design. Likewise, site feasibility, where the trial design is assessed in terms of whether a site can perform the trial as written and if both sites and subjects can be compliant with the protocol, is critical to assessing trial risk to understand how successful the trial may be.

Contract Research Organization (CRO)

CROs are specifically noted in the GCP guidelines – as they are a key partner in the conduct of clinical trials. A sponsor may transfer any or all of the sponsor's trial-related activities and functions to a CRO, but it is clear the sponsor retains ultimate accountability and responsibility for the activities. The CRO should be qualified and have a robust quality management system to guide their work, manage risk, and ensure quality. When transferring activities to a CRO, this should be specified in writing for both the sponsor and the CRO.

Implementation Tip – Prior to transferring activities to a CRO, a qualification audit must be performed to review processes, systems, and training to ensure the CRO (or any vendor) can work in a quality, compliant, and risk-focused manner. Sponsors should implement processes and procedures for vendor selection, qualification, and oversight to ensure appropriate criteria are applied to vendors who will perform trial activities on their behalf. When performing vendor qualification audits, the sponsor should apply their risk assessment criteria to determine the type and frequency of audit required to assess quality.

Implementation Tip – While CROs may perform the bulk of trial-related activities, it is critical that sponsors maintain written procedures (SOPs) and processes for those same procedures to provide adequate vendor oversight and monitoring of clinical trial work. The sponsor procedures are the ruler used to measure the performance of the CRO – even if the activities will follow the CRO SOPs for the trial.

Medical Expertise, Clinical Trial Design, and Data Handling

The sponsor should have appropriate medically qualified individuals available who can review and advise on trial-related medical queries or problems. This is important during the design and writing of the clinical trial protocol as well as throughout the conduct of the trial to review ongoing safety issues. As with all activities, qualified individuals representing key functions (safety, biostatistics, clinical supply, regulatory, data management, and clinical) should contribute to trial design and protocol development and all stages of trial execution.

It may be necessary in some trials for the sponsor to put an independent data-monitoring committee (IDMC) in place to assess the progress of the trial, safety data, and efficacy endpoints, as well as recommend whether the trial should be continued, modified, or stopped. These committees are critical to providing intended assessments of data to provide objectivity and help manage quality and risk.

When electronic systems are used for data capture and handling, it is the responsibility of the sponsor to ensure these systems are validated in a risk-appropriate manner, with appropriate security and safeguards in place to be compliant with applicable regulatory requirements. As electronic systems and data integrity are such critical issues in clinical trials, a chapter is dedicated to these key topics (see Chapter 11).

Investigator Selection

The selection of investigators to recruit subjects and medically treat them according to the clinical trial protocol is one of the most important activities in a trial. The sponsor is responsible for selecting qualified investigators with training and experience who can perform the requirements of the protocol. Investigators should be provided with the current clinical trial protocol as well as the Investigator's Brochure. Sponsors should ensure the investigator/institution agrees to conduct the trial in compliance with GCP and applicable regulatory requirements; agrees to data recording and reporting procedures; permits monitoring, auditing, and inspections; and will retain trial-related records for the specified document retention period. By signing and dating the protocol, the investigator confirms agreement with the above.

Implementation Tip – Sponsors should have a procedure for investigator selection and document their criteria for assessing investigator qualifications for each trial and the rationale for why specific investigators were chosen. This should be filed with trial-related documents as evidence for this activity during inspections.

Compensation to Subjects and Investigators and Other Financing

It is the responsibility of a sponsor to secure and provide insurance or indemnification against claims that may arise from the trial. Sponsors should adequately address the cost of treatment of trial subjects where trial-related injuries occur in line with applicable regulatory requirements.

Overall, an agreement should be in place for the financial aspects of the trial between the sponsor and investigator/institution.

Investigational Products

It is up to a sponsor to ensure there is adequate safety and efficacy data from nonclinical studies and/or clinical trials for safe human exposure as specified in the protocol design. This should be detailed in the current version of the Investigator's Brochure and updated with new information on a routine basis.

All investigational products, comparators, and placebos must be manufactured in accordance with accepted Good Manufacturing Practices (GMP). The labeling of these products should be appropriate for the clinical trial and any label blinding required for trial conduct. The storage, shipping, and stability conductions for the investigational product should be defined and monitored, and documentation should include safe and proper handling, reconstitution procedures, and any other specific instructions for use. In trials where the investigational product is blinded, a system that can rapidly decode the blind should be in place in case of a medical emergency. It is important to fully test and document the composition, stability, bioavailability, and other characteristics of the investigational product, especially when any changes are required or made, to ensure the product profile is fully characterized before use in a clinical trial.

Sponsors are responsible for supplying the investigative site with investigational products. Prior to the release of the product to an investigative site, the sponsor must perform a site initiation/regulatory green light visit to review and ensure essential documents are completed and in place, IRB/IEC approvals have been obtained, regulatory approval is granted (where required), contracts are in place, and required training is complete.

The accountability of all investigational products should be maintained by both the sponsor and the investigator/institution. This includes sponsor procedures for shipment and receipt of investigational material by the site and retrieval and/or destruction, as needed, during or at the end of a trial. The sponsor must also maintain procedures for retrieving investigational products as a result of safety or quality complaints or other issues that result in a product recall. Finally, ensuring the stability of the investigational product is the responsibility of the sponsor, and adequate quantities of the product must be available for the clinical trial.

Implementation Tip – Developing cross-functional procedures for clinical supplies will help to ensure a sponsor has an integrated approach to investigational products and clinical trials. This collaboration will streamline planning for trial logistics, ensure a timely trial start, and avoid disruptions related to investigational product delays.

Adverse Drug Reaction Reporting

If serious and unexpected adverse drug reactions (ADRs) occur during the course of a clinical trial, the sponsor is responsible for reporting these to all investigators/institutions, IRB/IECs, and regulatory authorities as required. This reporting (both expedited and annual/periodic updates) should align with local expedited reporting requirements and is further described in Chapter 10.

Monitoring

Monitoring clinical trial execution and data is a critical activity for the sponsor to undertake. The primary purpose is to ensure the rights and safety of subjects are protected, the trial data are accurate, verifiable, and complete, and the trial is conducted in adherence to an approved protocol, GCP, and local regulatory requirements.

Monitoring personnel are key partners who act on behalf of the sponsor directly with the investigator and site personnel. The sponsor should select monitors based on their qualifications and ability to adequately understand and ensure protocol compliance, the investigational product, informed consent, subject protections and safety, as well as sponsor procedures, GCP, and any regulatory requirements applicable to the trial.

Determining the level of monitoring required is a sponsor responsibility and should be aligned with and driven by the risk plan for the trial. By adopting a risk-based approach to monitoring – a balance of source data verification, on-site versus remote/centralized monitoring, and trial complexity –an adequate level of sponsor oversight is conducted to ensure the trial data meet the specified objectives, scientific endpoints, and regulatory compliance.

On-site monitoring is the most common approach, where all data and documents can be source-verified, drug accountability performed, and overall trial compliance assessed. With the growing use of electronic systems for trial data capture, there is more real-time data availability that lends itself to remote and/or centralized monitoring approaches. Regardless of the manner of monitoring utilized, the sponsor must outline their plan and rationale for the trial in a documented monitoring plan.

The monitor serves as the sponsor's main communication channel with the investigator and site personnel. For all monitoring visits, a standardized set of items should be reviewed, checked, confirmed, or collected as specified in the monitoring plan. This would include, at a minimum, confirming informed consent was granted for each subject, data review and querying of the case report forms (CRFs), dosing regimen, adverse event reporting, protocol adherence/deviations, investigative product accountability, and essential document review, among other routine assessments for compliance and adherence to GCP. For each visit, a written monitoring report should be generated, clearly recording all activities and reviews performed and any observations noted. The sponsor should review and approve these reports in a timely manner to ensure appropriate and controlled monitoring is occurring for a trial.

Implementation Tip – Sponsors should play an active role in developing a monitoring plan and actively review the ongoing monitoring activities performed by monitors. Active collaboration between sponsors and monitors is key to successful trial execution as is maintaining trial timelines and data quality standards.

Audits

The sponsor can and should perform periodic audits as a part of their quality assurance function to objectively assess qualifications, quality, ability to perform trial activities, and compliance with procedures, protocols, GCP, and any regulatory requirements that apply. Audits should be performed by independent experts who are qualified to assess the clinical trial or system being used. Sponsors should have a procedure for conducting audits (including risk assessment, frequency, scope, etc.) that is performed based on the importance of the clinical system/vendor being used or the criticality of the trial data being used for submission, and all audits should be documented in writing and maintained by the sponsor.

Noncompliance and Early Trial Termination or Suspension

In the event of noncompliance with procedures, protocols, GCP, or regulatory requirements, the sponsor must assess the noncompliance and determine if there is a significant impact on the trial outcome and data quality. If noncompliance impacts the wellbeing of the subject, it is important that a root cause analysis, corrective action, and preventive action plan be put into place. Depending on the risk posed by noncompliance, it may be necessary to remove the investigator from the trial. In that case, notification to the appropriate regulatory authorities and IRB/IEC may be required, especially if the noncompliance results in termination or suspension of the investigator.

Implementation Tip – Sponsors should be prepared for noncompliance occurrences by having a robust process to identify potential trial and investigator issues and immediately assess the safety and well-being of subjects impacted, but also determine the criticality of the issue, whether it impacts clinical trial data, the root cause of the noncompliance, and any corrective and preventive actions needed. Where serious breaches of trial conduct or patient safety are identified, reporting to the appropriate regulatory agency may be required.

CLINICAL TRIAL PROTOCOL AND PROTOCOL AMENDMENTS

The clinical trial protocol is a central document for the description of the trial, the rationale of the study, and what it entails for trial subjects and investigative sites. While the trial design should be customized for the product being investigated, there are key sections that should be included in each protocol:

- **General Information** – Including title, protocol number, date, amendment number (as appropriate), name and contact information of the sponsor, monitoring partner, sponsor medical expert, qualified physician or dentist for site-related medical (dental) decisions, and clinical laboratories or other medical services or institutions used in the trial. In addition, it should include signatures for the sponsor and investigator.
- **Background Information** – This section should include the name and description of the investigational product, a summary of the nonclinical study findings that have potential clinical significance, and any previous clinical trial data that is relevant. The known potential risks and benefits should be summarized. This section should include a description and justification for the route of administration, dosage, regimen, and treatment period. A statement should be included that the trial will be conducted in compliance with the protocol, GCP, and applicable regulatory requirements. A description of the population to be studied should be present in this section. Relevant literature and data should also be noted.
- **Trial Objective and Purpose** – In this section, a detailed description of the objectives and purpose of the trial should be stated.
- **Trial Design** – The protocol should include a detailed description of the clinical trial design. This description supports the scientific integrity of the trial and the credibility of the data. The description of the trial design should include:
  - Statement of primary and secondary endpoints to be measured;
  - Description of the type/design of the trial (e.g., double-blind, placebo-controlled, parallel design) with an accompanying visual outlining the design, procedures, and stages;
  - Measures taken to minimize and avoid bias, including randomization and blinding, if required;
  - Trial treatments, dosage, and dosage regimen, including dosing form, packaging, and labeling of the investigational product;
  - Expected duration of subject participation with a description of the sequence and duration of the trial periods and follow-ups;
  - Criteria for stopping or disconsolation for individual subjects and/or parts of the trial or entire trial;
  - Accountability procedures for the investigational product, placebo, and comparator(s), if any;
  - The mechanism for maintaining treatment randomization codes and the process for breaking codes;
  - Data to be recorded directly into the CRFs, where this data becomes the source data.
- **Selection and Withdrawal of Subjects** – the inclusion and exclusion criteria for the trial should be detailed, as should the subject withdrawal criteria and procedures.
- **Treatment of Subjects** – a detailed description of the treatments that will be administered, including name, doses, dosing schedule, route of administration, treatment and follow-up periods, other medications/treatments that

are permitted (including rescue medications, as appropriate) or those that are specifically excluded during the clinical trial period, and the procedures for ensuring the subject's compliance.

- **Assessment of Efficacy** – a description of the efficacy parameters and how they will be assessed, measured, and analyzed.
- **Assessment of Safety** – a description of the safety parameters for the trial, including the procedure for recording and reporting adverse events and the required follow-up.
- **Statistics** – the statistical methods to be used for any analyses (interim and final) should be described. It should also include the number of subjects to be enrolled, and a rationale for the sample size to justify the power of the statistical analysis. Criteria for the termination of the trial and procedures for handling the data should be specified.
- **Direct Access to Source Data/Documents** – it is important that the investigator/institution knows that direct access to trial-related data/documents and monitoring, and IRB/IEC review, is required, and audits and possible regulatory inspections should be supported by the investigator.
- Quality Control and Quality Assurance
- **Ethics** – a description of ethical considerations incorporated in the trial design and conduct.
- Data Handling and Record Keeping
- **Financing and Insurance** – include in the protocol if not incorporated into a separate site agreement.
- **Publication Policy** – include in the protocol if not incorporated into a separate site agreement.
- **Supplements** – include any supplemental information necessary to help inform the investigator.

Implementation Tip To support quality across clinical development programs, sponsors should adopt a standard company template for clinical trial protocols that incorporates the key components outlined above. In addition, implementing a standard procedure for developing a protocol, including cross-functional involvement, review, and approval, will contribute to mitigating the risks associated with the trial and provide thoughtful insights into the design and conduct of the trial and across trials.

INVESTIGATOR'S BROCHURE

For an investigator to fully understand the investigational product being used for a clinical trial, sponsors create an Investigator's Brochure (IB), which is a compilation of the nonclinical and clinical data accumulated on the product in humans. This will instruct the investigator on the rationale for the use of the product, its mode of action, route of administration, dosing, and other key clinical factors that can impact the treatment of subjects. The information presented should be clear, concise, objective, balanced, and non-promotional in nature to ensure the investigator can make the most informed decisions possible about treatment for the subject.

The focus of the IB will change over the course of clinical development. For early trials, it will be more heavily weighted with nonclinical data. As clinical information, especially safety data, becomes available, the IB is updated to include this new information. To ensure the IB is up to date it should be reviewed and updated at least annually, and more often if relevant new information can impact the safety and treatment of subjects.

The IB should include the following sections:

- **Title Page** – includes sponsor name, investigational product name/number, chemical name, trade name, release date, IB version number and date.
- **Confidentiality Statement** – this is a reminder that the IB is a confidential document and is a key resource for the investigator and IRB/IEC.
- Table of Contents
- **Summary** – a brief overview (not more than two pages), describing the important physical, chemical, pharmaceutical, pharmacological, toxicological, pharmacokinetic, metabolic, and clinical information available that is relevant to the stage of clinical development.
- Introduction
- **Physical, Chemical, and Pharmaceutical Properties and Formulation** – This section covers the chemical structure and properties of the investigational product as well as safe handling, storage, and dosing of the product.
- Nonclinical Studies
    - **Introduction** – The results of relevant nonclinical studies should be described in a manner (tabular, where possible) that outlines the relevance of these findings to the therapy, and any unfavorable or unintended effects in humans.
    - **Nonclinical Pharmacology** – An overview of the pharmacological aspects of the investigational product and an assessment of its potential therapeutic activity
    - **Pharmacokinetics and Product Metabolism in Animals** – A discussion of the findings addressing the adsorption and local and systemic bioavailability of the investigational product and its metabolites.
    - **Toxicology** – Includes a summary of the toxicological effects found in the studies and describes (where appropriate) the effects of single doses, repeated doses, carcinogenicity, special studies, reproductive toxicity, and genotoxicity.
- Effects on Humans
    - **Introduction** – T his section should contain a complete discussion of the known effects of the investigational product on humans. If clinical trials have been completed, a summary of results should be provided as well, or if marketed, any pertinent information related to the product.
    - **Pharmacokinetics and Product Metabolism in Humans** – An overall summary of pharmacokinetics, bioavailability, population subgroups, interactions, and other pharmacokinetic data.
    - **Safety and Efficacy** – This section highlights and discusses the safety profile of the investigational product, supported by data from clinical

trials already performed. As new data is obtained, this section will be updated to describe possible risks and adverse drug reactions that are anticipated based on prior experiences.

- **Marketing Experience** – For products that may be marketed or approved in some countries, this should be listed in the IB. Any findings of significance that have arisen from marketed use should be summarized. If an investigational product did not gain marketing approval or was withdrawn from a market, that would also be noted in the IB.

- **Summary of Data and Guidance for the Investigator** – This provides the investigator with an overall summary of the nonclinical and clinical data to enable the most informed decision making for subjects. It should be made very clear how the product works and the potential risks and adverse reactions that may occur. In addition, guidance on the recognition and treatment of possible overdoses and adverse reactions should be described.

Implementation Tip – One challenge many companies have is identifying the functional owner of the IB. It is important to define who is accountable for the initial IB development as well as the annual reviews and updates. Implementing a cross-functional process with defined timelines, standardized templates, and review and approval cycles will lead to a more robust and quality IB.

ESSENTIAL DOCUMENTS FOR THE CONDUCT OF A CLINICAL TRIAL

Essential documents are a collection of key documents that provide evidence of how the trial was conducted by the sponsor and the investigator as well as supporting the quality of the data generated from the clinical trial. The purpose of these documents is to demonstrate the sponsor, investigator, and monitor's adherence to GCP and any applicable regulatory requirements.

The value of producing and filing essential documents in a timely manner is that it can help facilitate the smooth conduct of the trial by all parties involved. These are also the documents that are routinely monitored throughout the trial and are key items for audits and inspections to confirm the trial data is valid and the trial was conducted with integrity.

To assist the sponsor, monitors, and investigators with managing essential documents, the list has been divided into three sections based on the order in which they will be generated: (i) before the clinical trial commences (prior to subject enrollment), (ii) during the conduct of the trial, and (iii) after the completion of the trial – and whether the document is to be filed with the Investigator/Institution or the Sponsor.

A trial master file (TMF) should be established by both the sponsor and investigator (the TMF at the investigative site is often referred to as an Investigator Site File (ISF)) at the beginning of the trial. These files will be updated throughout the course of the trial and should be monitored throughout. It is important to remember that all essential documents may be audited and inspected at any time; therefore, it is important that these records are current, correct, and complete. Regardless of the method by which the TMF/ISF is documented (e.g., paper, electronic, or a combination of both), a process should be in place for maintaining source documents, long-term storage, and document identification, versioning, searching, and retrieval. For some trials, it may be appropriate to add to or reduce the essential document set based on the design or requirements of the trial. This should be done prior to the trial starting and documented in writing at that time.

The sponsor should always ensure the investigator has access to and control of the CRF data for the trial, even when in an electronic system. In addition, the investigator should have control of all essential documents that are generated by the investigator.

The list of essential documents can be found in ICH E6(R2), section 8.2 (Before the Clinical Phase of the Trial Commences); section 8.3 (During the Clinical Conduct of the Trial); and section 8.4 (After Completion or Termination of the Trial). It is good practice to always refer directly to the regulation to ensure compliance with the requirement.

CONCLUSION

GCP is designed to provide standardized guidance for sponsors and investigators to design and conduct clinical trials that focus on the generation of high-quality data while ensuring the protection of human subjects. GCP provides the framework for implementing quality standards by sponsors and investigators before, as they conduct, and after the closure of trial activities. While GCP is the minimum standard required, sponsors and investigators should carefully consider how they will implement and build on this guidance to best provide for the well-being of subjects.

There are efforts in progress to further modernize GCP and integrate it with other standards of quality, and this will be further discussed in Chapter 4. Even with future changes, the guiding principles of GCP remain the same – ensuring the rights, safety, and general well-being of subjects are protected while generating quality, reliable data.

NOTES

1 How the thalidomide scandal led to safer drugs. James Kingsland. Medical News Today, December 15, 2020. https://www.medicalnewstoday.com/articles/how-the-thalidomide-scandal-led-to-safer-drugs
2 Integrated Addendum to ICH E6(R1): Guideline for Good Clinical Practice E6(R2), Current Step 4 version, dated 9 November 2016. https://database.ich.org/sites/default/files/E6_R2_Addendum.pdf
3 Integrated Addendum to ICH E6(R1): Guideline for Good Clinical Practice E6(R2), Current Step 4 version, dated 9 November 2016. https://database.ich.org/sites/default/files/E6_R2_Addendum.pdf
4 E6(R2) Good Clinical Practice: Integrated Addendum to ICH E6(R1) Guidance for Industry, March 2018. https://www.fda.gov/media/93884/download
5 The Principles of ICH GCP, Section 2.1.
6 Sponsor Quality Management, Section 5.0; Integrated Addendum to ICH E6(R1): Guideline for Good Clinical Practice E6(R2), Current Step 4 version, dated 9 November 2016. https://database.ich.org/sites/default/files/E6_R2_Addendum.pdf

3 Quality by Design, Critical to Quality Factors – ICH E8(R1)

Sandra "Sam" Sather and Jennifer Lawyer

INTRODUCTION

Clinical trial design and conduct have become more complex, impacting the time and cost required to develop medicinal products. The International Council for Harmonisation (ICH) "E8(R1) General Considerations for Clinical Studies" (ICH, 2021a; FDA, 2022) was developed to address concerns about the principles of trial design and planning that are needed to ensure an appropriate level of data quality. The revision incorporates current concepts, including fit-for-purpose data quality, as one of the essential considerations for all clinical trials. It expands the idea of a proportionate approach to trial design and conduct and the process of focusing on the items that are critical to the quality of the study – the protection of study participants and the reliability of the data – to ensure that the results are quality enough to support good decision-making. The focus is not on the perfection of results but on the assurance of quality.

The main areas of quality consideration in the revised guideline are as follows:

- Quality by Design (QbD), or designing quality into the protocol and processes
- Focusing on Critical to Quality (CtQ) factors using a risk-proportionate approach
- Establishing a framework to identify and review CtQ factors
- Utilizing multiple sources of data to support the CtQ factors, including real-world data, where permitted
- Establishing a culture that supports open dialog using critical thinking and risk-based prioritization for building QbD
- Paying careful attention to design elements and collecting only data that link to the CtQ factors.

BACKGROUND

ICH E8 had not been revised since it was first adopted in 1997. The focus of the April 2022 revision is to modernize clinical trial design, planning, management, conduct, and reporting. Note that the main concepts overlap with ICH E6 GCP (Good Clinical Practice), which was a purposeful laying of the foundation for the ICH E6

DOI: 10.1201/9781003407010-3

Renovation. The 1997 Guideline focused on simple protocol design and single-site clinical trials that were likely academic and that used paper data sources. Originally, the guideline used the term "drug" to mean all investigational products, including devices, but the focus in the revision is on medicinal products. This is because ISO standards are followed for global medical device GCP (such as ISO 13485 Medical devices – Quality management systems – Requirements for regulatory purposes; ISO 14155:2020 GCP medical devices; ISO 14971:2019 Application of Risk Management to medical devices), many of which have been updated and modernized recently.

ICH E8 can be thought of as the "master" guideline to map to the entire ICH E family, including ICH E6(R3), Good Clinical Practice. The 'E' family of guidelines is interrelated and should be read together. The key focus of ICH E8(R1) is to design quality into clinical trials, or QbD , which is supported by the establishment of an appropriate framework for the identification and review of CtQ factors at the time of design and planning of the study, and throughout its conduct, analysis, and reporting.

The GCP renovation began with the 2017 ICH Reflection Paper soon after ICH E6(R2) was finalized (ICH 2017, 2016). The Reflection Paper was further revised in 2021 (ICH, 2021b). It identified gaps in the E8 and E6(R2) guidelines. Even before the Reflection Paper, there was a push within ICH to modernize pretty much all of their guidelines. ICH E6(R2) was not flexible enough for the way modern clinical trials are conducted. Clinical trials became more complicated, with larger amounts of data and more complex protocols that needed a more scalable and adaptive approach. Additionally, there is a greater use of digital media and technologies, an increased emphasis on risk-based quality management, and the rise of non-traditional and innovative clinical trial design, including the use of real-world data and consulting patients who have the condition being studied. These were not anticipated or adequately discussed in the original guidelines. Having a good understanding of how to utilize the varied methods of modern clinical trial planning, conduct, and reporting while retaining quality became more important.

Areas where there was a great deal of change which was identified for the ICH E8 revision, as described in the GCP Reflection Paper, include:

- the wide range of clinical trial designs and data sources that are currently used in drug development;
- approaches for optimizing clinical trial quality, which promote the reliability, efficiency, and patient focus of clinical trials;
- a focus on identifying the factors that are critical to the quality of a clinical trial early enough at the design stage; and
- planning the study conduct proportionate to the risks to these CtQ factors.

DATA QUALITY AND QBD

ICH E8(R1) is intended to address concerns about the principles of trial design and planning that are needed to ensure an appropriate level of data quality. Quality occurs when there are the right answers to the scientific questions to support decision-making while protecting study participants. The revised guideline includes a review of the issues and questions that are most critical to clinical trial quality and the ability of a trial to achieve meaningful and reliable results. Additionally, E8(R1) incorporates the current Guidelines for achieving fit-for-purpose data quality as one of the essential considerations for all clinical trials, including the broad range of designs and data sources currently in use.

QbD is linked to continuous improvement. The organization should identify what metrics would measure the outcomes of QbD implementation to guide updates to process improvements that are linked to the CtQ factors. For example, metrics that would measure important risks, study participant enrollment and early terminations, major and critical audit observations, important protocol deviations, etc. To measure the effectiveness of the implementation of QbD, a maturity model can be used. An example is CTTI Quality by Design Maturity Model, which outlines five maturity levels (Ad hoc, Early, Developing, Implementing, and Optimizing) across four main factors: (i) Quality Culture, (ii) Study Design, (iii) Study Conduct, and (iv) Continuous Improvement for organizations to identify where they are now and what the goals are for growth (CTTI Quality by Design (QbD) Maturity Model, 2023).

RISK MANAGEMENT

There is an increased focus on the importance of identifying a set of factors CtQ and risks that would threaten quality. Quality is based on good study design and execution, and quality studies protect study participants, ensure the integrity of data, and manage risks. Quality is fit for purpose, which for clinical trials means data that are reliable to answer the research questions and support decision-making while protecting study participants (ICH E8(R1) Section 2.2). Keep in mind that the focus of change is on improved quality and is not just a time- and money-saving activity. Organizational changes must occur from the top down, starting with senior leadership. With the change in mindset, organizations should ensure team members are supported and rewarded for using critical thinking and risk-based prioritization.

The revised guideline cautions that a risk-based approach is frequently burdened by an overly complex study design. A risk-proportionate approach to study design necessitates a focus on only the data that are CtQ. Just because additional visits or lab results might be interesting to study, if they do not directly support critical safety or endpoint data, consider if they are really necessary or if they may be overly burdensome for clinical sites, study participants, as well as sponsor or CRO monitors, data management, etc.

Unlike in ICH E6(R2) in section 5.0, which places the responsibility of risk-based quality management on the sponsor, the E8(R1) Guideline expands this to other stakeholders including clinical sites and ethics committees. There is a need to customize the design based on the specific needs of each study, not by using a one-size-fits-all approach. Risk management links to QbD, where risks can be anticipated and study design is adaptable. The approach determines if impacts are acceptable or how to mitigate risks if not. It focuses efforts on elements that are essential to study participant protection and outcomes that are meaningful to the participants while seeking stakeholders' input to inform the study design. Lastly, it is anticipated that stakeholders will review and modify identified risks and risk management plans as needed.

CONSIDERATIONS FOR DETERMINING CTQ FACTORS

The revised guideline provides a basic set of CtQ factors that can be adapted to different types of clinical trials, including traditional or adaptive design. A result of the CtQ factors would be to have more meaningful eligibility criteria, statistical analysis, and so on. Another goal is to address a broader range of clinical trial designs and data sources, including electronic. Lastly, it provides an updated comprehensive guide that cross-references all other relevant ICH Guidelines without reproducing the detailed material found in those guidelines. Note that identifying everything in a clinical trial as critical is neither feasible nor desirable and would overburden the process. Following QbD by using a risk-based approach to select which elements are CtQ is imperative. A QbD approach involves the identification of CtQ factors that should be supported by proactive, cross-functional discussions and decision-making at the time of study planning. Different factors will stand out as critical for different types of studies, following the concepts introduced throughout the guideline.

The goal of a QbD approach is to focus attention on the design of all components of the study protocol, procedures, and associated operational plans. This will ensure the likelihood that a study will answer the research questions posed reliably and meaningfully for decision-makers and individuals with the studied condition while preventing critical errors. Following a QbD approach decreases the overreliance on retrospective document checking, monitoring, auditing, or inspection and is instead more proactive.

Considerations for identifying CtQ factors that need to be integrated into the culture of the organization for effective decision-making and to ensure a quality study are listed in Section 7 of the revised guideline.

- Stakeholder Engagement
- Non-clinical Data Support
- Study Objectives
- Meaningful Comparison to Control
- Protection of Study Participants
- Information to Study Participants
- Training
- Feasibility
- Study Participants, Duration, and Frequency of Visits
- Eligibility Criteria
- Data Collection per Protocol
- Response Variables
- Reduce Bias
- Statistical Analysis Plan
- Data Integrity
- Monitoring
- Data Monitoring Committee
- Report of Study Results

Note that at different points in the development of the medicinal product, new information informs the identification of CtQ factors and the control processes used to manage them.

CTQ CONTINUES

Concern for CtQ does not end with the database lock. CtQ factors should be a consideration for regulatory submissions and continued inspection readiness until marketing approval. CtQ factors for inspection readiness are topics that are linked to data reliability and study participant safety and rights. These would be processes that link to safety data, primary and secondary endpoints, and other critical processes that really matter. Regulatory authorities focus inspection activities on quality oversight of all aspects of the clinical trial. With the ICH E8(R1) focus on the CtQ factors for the study design, building quality into the design with periodic review and utilizing risk-based quality management to detect if changes are needed is the first step in being inspection-ready. For continued inspection readiness, map the CtQ factors determined for the specifics of the study to the history of what really happened. Using the CtQ approach, focus on where to be prepared to speak to the regulatory authority regarding:

- Were there processes in place for the quality of the study?
- Were the processes followed?
- If the processes were not followed, what was done to ensure quality?

In addition, the information gathered through the inspection readiness activities can inform proactive process improvement in other programs and at an organization level for continued adaptation of a QbD approach with the ultimate goal of moving upwards in the Maturity Model.

CONCLUSION

The modernization of ICH E8 was the first step towards the Renovation of Good Clinical Practice that began in 2017. The revision incorporates CtQ factors as one of the essential considerations for all clinical trials. It expands the idea of a proportionate approach to clinical trial design and conduct and the process of focusing on the protection of study participants and the reliability of the results, or other processes that support what really matters, in an effort to ultimately ensure that the results are of high quality to support a marketing application. The focus is not on the perfection of results but on the assurance of quality through a careful selection of CtQ factors, utilizing proactive QbD with a risk-proportionate approach, and supporting critical thinking throughout the organization.

REFERENCES

CTTI Quality by Design (QbD) Maturity Model (2023). Clinical Trials Transformation Initiative. Retrieved 24Nov2023. URL https://ctti-clinicaltrials.org/wp-content/uploads/2023/05/CTTI_QbD_Maturity_Model.pdf

FDA (2022). *Guidance for Industry: E8(R1) General Considerations for Clinical Studies.* U.S. Department of Health and Human Services, Food and Drug Administration, Center for Drug Evaluation and Research (CDER), Center for Biologics Evaluation and Research (CBER). Revised April 2022.

ICH (2016). *ICH Harmonised Guideline: Integrated Addendum to ICH E6(R1): Guideline for Good Clinical Practice E6(R2).* International Council for Harmonisation. 9 November 2016.

ICH (2017). ICH Reflection on "GCP Renovation": Modernization of ICH E8 and Subsequent Renovation of ICH E6. International Council for Harmonisation. Revised January 2017. ICH (2021a). *ICH Harmonised Guideline: E8(R1) General Considerations for Clinical Studies.* International Council for Harmonisation. 6 October 2021.

ICH (2021b). *ICH Reflection on "GCP Renovation": Modernization of ICH E8 and Subsequent Renovation of ICH E6.* International Council for Harmonisation. Revised May 2021.

4 Good Clinical Practice – Modernizing ICH E6

John S. Klein, Sonya T. Edgerton, and Sandra "Sam" Sather

INTRODUCTION

As the life sciences industry evolves, the products they create are ever more complex and innovative. To adequately ensure these products are safe and effective, the clinical trials needed have become more complex. In addition, the technology available to capture data has expanded to match the needs of the 21st century. With all this innovation and growth, the principles that govern clinical trial conduct also need to evolve and grow to meet the current and future needs of the industry. While the rights and safety of trial subjects must continue to be at the forefront of any changes, new concepts about how we conduct clinical trials can lead to a better, more integrated approach to clinical trial design and execution.

ICH E6(R2) became the global standard for how clinical trials are conducted; however, to better meet the needs of an evolving industry, a Good Clinical Practice (GCP) renovation is needed to change the mindset of those who conduct trials to better focus on protecting human participants and improving data quality. The new renovated approach is to create a mindset of quality – one that brings the various components of International Council for Harmonization (ICH) guidelines into a cohesive and integrated approach for conducting clinical trials. This chapter will focus on the key changes to ICH E6 that are known as ICH E6(R3) Draft Guideline currently under consideration. These general concepts have received widespread endorsement but are still under review and finalization as of this writing.

HOLISTIC THINKING FOR CLINICAL TRIAL DESIGN AND EXECUTION

At the forefront, clinical trials must be designed and conducted with the rights and well-being of the trial subjects (now called trial participants in ICH E6(R3)) protected. This is the most important consideration and should be the focus of every component of trial design and conduct.

One of the key principles this modernization effort seeks to achieve is to better integrate the different components of the ICH guidelines. To this end, we see more references to components of the guidelines that are interrelated. This is important, as the various guidelines address key areas for collaborative consideration by sponsors and investigators. For example, ICH E8(R1), covered in detail in Chapter 3,

DOI: 10.1201/9781003407010-4

discusses Quality by Design and Critical to Quality Factors in clinical trials. These concepts are indispensable to designing and conducting clinical trials with quality as an underlying foundation that minimizes risk, focuses on the safety of trial participants, and leads to better trial design and outcomes. Modernization of the guidelines is also intended to support a broader range of trial designs and approaches and to encourage thoughtful consideration and planning to address the unique aspects of individual clinical trials. The revision to ICH E8 was a key step to modernize the approach to quality in clinical trials. Now that ICH E8(R1) is in place, it paves the way for the updates to ICH E6(R2) to better support unique trials and data sources.

The changes proposed in ICH E6(R3) are designed to be more open-ended to allow for more flexibility in trial design and execution. This increased flexibility aims to encourage reflective thinking on how risks and participants' safety can be optimized without reducing trial activities to mere checklists that must be completed.

The modernized approach also brings new focus to how the sponsor and investigator collaborate on their respective responsibilities and interactions throughout the design and conduct of a trial. Thoughtfulness in trial design and conduct, fit-for-purpose approaches, incorporating lessons learned from other innovatively designed trials and past experiences are all built into the fabric of ICH E6(R3).

A core concept focuses on trial and data reproducibility. Where data integrity remains a critical factor, the quality and reproducibility of the data are integrated into the approach. To this end, modernization embraces the wide range of real-world data that is available to inform decision-making in trial design and conduct. In addition to available data, the increased role of technology (e.g., electronic documentation, electronic signatures) available in clinical trials should be embraced and adopted.

INSTITUTIONAL REVIEW BOARD/INDEPENDENT ETHICS COMMITTEE (IRB/IEC)

The overriding purpose of the IRB/IEC is to protect the rights, safety, and well-being of trial participants. To that end, the IRB/IEC is responsible for the ethical review of a trial and should conduct its work in conjunction with applicable local regulatory requirements. The work of the IRB/IEC is to review and endorse the clinical trial protocol, informed consent and assent forms, the Investigator's Brochure, and any other information that is provided to trial participants.

A new section in ICH E6(R3) for the IRB/IEC is that of Submission and Communication. Where submissions and communications with the IRB/IEC are also required to be made to relevant regulatory authorities, these may be combined, where applicable, to streamline submissions.

INVESTIGATOR

The investigator (and/or the institution) is expected to take a greater role in oversight and responsibility for the work done on their behalf (either by their personnel or a suitable service provider). There should be clear roles and responsibilities and delegation of trial-related activities. The investigator's compliance with the protocol remains a key requirement and deviations from the protocol must be documented and reported to the sponsor, IRB/IEC, and/or regulatory authorities as required. Safety reporting requirements by the investigator are also clearly established as defined in the clinical trial protocol.

Investigators and sites must take a risk-based approach to quality management. Doing so should include a timely review of data, including external data sources. The investigator's role in quality and risk mitigation cannot be understated.

Informed Consent

As with ICH E6(R2), the consent requirements are listed in some detail, with some new caveats. Informed consent should be obtained and documented in paper or electronic (eConsent) format, ensuring adherence to GCP and other ethical principles to protect participants. Consent must be given willingly, must be clear, and must be in an understandable native language. ICH E6(R3) contains additional details surrounding the requirements and situations where a participant's legally acceptable representative can be involved in the consent process and provide consent. Assent is a new term in ICH E6(R3) that documents the affirmative agreement of a minor to participate in a clinical trial. When a minor is included as a trial participant, there must be age-appropriate assent information provided to the minor, and assent must be obtained prior to enrollment.

Records

The investigator has a responsibility for generating, recording, and reporting trial data and should ensure the integrity of the data they are responsible for providing. ICH E6(R3) includes more rigorous data governance that details expanded requirements for the investigator that include:

- Avoiding unnecessary transcription steps;
- Timely review of data (including from external sources) that may impact the eligibility, treatment, or safety of the participant;
- Ensuring data are collected and systems are used as intended;
- Endorsing reported data at milestones agreed upon with the sponsor;
- When using computerized systems, adequately managing access, training participants, and reporting incidents to the sponsor;
- Addressing and implementing the measures outlined in the section on data governance proportionately for systems deployed by the investigator/institution for clinical trial purposes.

SPONSOR

The sponsor remains responsible for implementing risk-proportionate processes to ensure the safety of trial participants and the reliability of trial results throughout the entire clinical trial lifecycle. It is incumbent on sponsors to design trials in a way that incorporates prior data (nonclinical and clinical) as well as real-world data where possible. They must also incorporate quality into the design of the trial by proactively identifying the factors that are critical to quality for the trial and managing those risk factors. In designing clinical trials, sponsors should gather input from a wide variety of stakeholders, including healthcare professionals and patients, to meet the expectations outlined in ICH E8(R1) for both the protocol and the informed consent materials. Finally, sponsors should ensure that clinical trials are operationally feasible and avoid unnecessary complexity, procedures, and data collection. To this end, clinical trials should be fit for purpose.

Agreements

Agreements that the sponsor makes with investigators/institutions, service providers, and any other parties that are involved with the clinical trial are to be documented prior to beginning those activities. They must indicate that the investigator/institution or service provider will conduct the work in accordance with the approved protocol and in compliance with GCP and local regulatory requirements. Where the responsibilities of the sponsor are transferred to or assumed by a service provider, they must be documented in writing. Regardless of activities transferred, the sponsor retains ultimate responsibility for all trial-related activities, participant safety, and trial data. The sponsor must have processes for selecting, assessing, and overseeing all trial-related activities transferred to and performed by service providers.

Sponsor Oversight

The sponsor has the ultimate responsibility to ensure the trial design and conduct, processes, and data generated are of a high level of quality to ensure the reliability of trial results, the participant's safety, and adequate decision-making. To further support this, sponsors will need to proactively classify protocol deviations that are important (those impacting participants rights, safety, and well-being, or impacting trial results reliability) through trial-specific criteria.

Sponsor oversight should be fit for purpose and match the complexity and risk profile of the trial. This includes the selection and oversight of investigators and service providers. There must be an issue escalation process that ensures timely assessment and implementation of actions to mitigate risk and ensure quality.

Quality Management

The sponsor must implement a quality system that manages quality throughout the clinical trial lifecycle and process. The purpose is to ensure the participants' well-being and safety, and the trial results are reliable and repeatable. There is a more direct link to ICH E8(R1) with this update that ties the two guidelines together in a more seamless manner. Quality must be built into all components of a clinical trial, and the sponsor should describe the quality management approach they used in the clinical trial report (linked to ICH E3).

Risk control and mitigation are important parts of quality management. Risk mitigation may be incorporated into all aspects of a trial – including protocol design and conduct, monitoring plans, agreements, ensuring SOPs are followed, and training content. Ongoing assessment of the risks present in a trial, with appropriate actions and documented plans to mitigate them, will become a standard part of clinical trial conduct. Where risk cannot be mitigated, it must be controlled to an acceptable level proportionate to the degree of risk and impact on the trial.

Quality Assurance and Quality Control

The sponsor remains responsible for establishing, implementing, and maintaining appropriate quality assurance and quality control processes and documented procedures to ensure trials are conducted in compliance with protocols and GCP/regulatory requirements. The audit requirements remain unchanged and should be done proportionate to the level of risk associated with the conduct of the trial.

Quality control extends beyond sites and service providers to each stage of data handling to ensure data are reliable and have been properly processed. Monitoring and data management processes are key quality control activities in a trial. For site monitoring, quality control may include on-site and/or centralized monitoring activities that may be used to fulfill the defined risk-based approach for the trial.

Monitoring encompasses a wide range of activities fundamentally designed to protect and ensure participants' rights, safety, and well-being, as well as the reliability of trial results throughout the conduct of the trial. Approaches to monitoring should consider all the various activities and services involved in trial conduct, including on-site and decentralized settings, and should be detailed in a monitoring plan. It is critical that monitors and trial staff consider data protection and confidentiality at the forefront of their work. The extent and nature of monitoring activities should be appropriate and risk-based and documented in the monitoring plan and include source data review and an appropriate level of source data verification (SDV). Where various monitoring methods and tools are used, the rationale and risks associated with their use should be detailed in the monitoring plan.

Monitoring activities, as defined by the sponsor's requirements and the monitoring plan, should include communication with parties conducting the trial, selecting investigator sites, conducting site initiation, ongoing trial management and close-out activities, investigational product management, monitoring of clinical trial data, and documenting and summarizing all monitoring activities in a monitoring report. The sponsor maintains responsibility for monitoring performance, oversight, and governance throughout the conduct of the clinical trial. As required, the sponsor should conduct audits in alignment with their approved audit process.

Safety Assessment and Reporting

This expanded requirement places more emphasis on the sponsor's review of safety information throughout the trial. This review may result in new data that can impact a participant's willingness to continue participation in the trial, how the trial is conducted, or the ongoing approval of an IRB/IEC or regulatory authorities. The sponsor is responsible for submitting safety updates and periodic reports to the appropriate regulatory authorities which may include required changes to the Investigator's

Brochure. Expedited safety reporting is required for all adverse drug reactions (ADRs) that are suspected, unexpected, and serious (SUSARs), as described in ICH E2A (and further detailed in Chapter 5).

Safety reporting should also assess the expectedness of a reaction as it relates to the applicable product information (for example, the reference safety information (RSI) found in the Investigator's Brochure). Where urgency or reporting is required, reporting of SUSARs should occur to the investigator/institutions, and IRB/IEC in a manner that reflects the urgency. Should an immediate hazard exist or a serious breach occur, sponsors should take prompt action to mitigate the hazard/breach and inform all parties impacted.

Data and Records

This revised section covers Data Handling, Statistical Programming and Data Analysis, Record Keeping and Retention, and Record Access. This section adds focus to the sponsor's need to ensure the integrity and confidentiality of data that is generated and managed in a clinical trial. To this end, the sponsor should:

- Pre-specify the data to be collected and a data overview.
- Provide guidance for the investigator/institutions, service providers, and trial participants, as needed, on the expectations for data capture, data changes, data retention, and data disposal.
- Ensure the investigator has access to the data collected, including relevant external data, for the full retention period.
- Seek investigator endorsement of their data at pre-determined milestones.

In addition to applying quality controls to data handling and management, sponsors should ensure the tools used for data acquisition are fit for purpose and designed to capture the information required by the protocol. The sponsor should also ensure tools and systems are validated and ready for use prior to their use in a trial. Documented processes should support the implementation and use of these tools to ensure data integrity throughout the data life cycle, and adequate training on these tools should be available for users.

Documentation of the data management steps that will be utilized should be in place prior to any data analysis activities. This applies to data that will be used for an Independent Data Monitoring Committee (IDMC) or any analysis conducted (interim or final). Deviations from the approved steps should be documented accordingly.

There is an expanded requirement for computer system validation for any tools or systems used in a clinical trial – both by the sponsor and those utilized by the investigative site. All tools should be assessed, and the validation status should be known during site selection, and this should be documented.

To bridge the gap between ICH E6(R2) and ICH E9 (Statistical Principles for Clinical Trials), there is an expanded section on Statistical Programming and Data Analysis in this updated guidance. This includes requiring the sponsor to have appropriate and documented quality control over statistical programming and data analysis. Robust processes for statistical programming and data analysis must be ensured by the sponsor as well. In addition, the sponsor must also document and justify deviations from the planned statistical analysis or changes made to the analysis data set after the trial has been unblinded. Procedures should be in place to cover aspects of unblinding and document occurrences of unblinding. It is incumbent on the sponsor to retain statistical records that are used in the reporting of trial results, including the quality control and validation activities utilized. The traceability of data and data sources must ensure that data can be traced back to the original data. Once reported, results should be retained in a non-editable format.

The sections on Record Keeping and Retention and that of Record Access bring together key requirements the sponsor has for maintaining records. This streamlines the requirements into the same section and makes it easier for sponsors to comply with the requirements in their jurisdiction.

DATA GOVERNANCE – INVESTIGATOR AND SPONSOR

A new section in ICH E6(R3) covers data governance for both the investigators and the sponsors. The goal here is to provide integrated guidance for data integrity, traceability, and security to support accurate reporting, verification, and interpretation of clinical trial results and information throughout the data life cycle. This should be considered by both investigators and sponsors in alignment with ICH E8(R1) and ICH E9. The updated section reiterates the need to design and implement systems and processes in a way that is proportionate to the risks to participants and trial result reliability. The key processes needed to address the full data life cycle and focus on the criticality of data should be implemented proportionately with the appropriate documentation:

- *Processes to ensure the protection of trial participants' confidential data;*
- *Process for managing computerized systems to ensure they are fit for purpose and used appropriately;*
- *Processes to safeguard essential elements of the clinical trial (randomization, dose escalation, blinding);*
- *Processes to support key decision-making, such as finalization prior to analysis, unblinding, allocation of analysis data sets, changes in clinical trial design, and IDMC, where applicable (Reference: ICH E6(R3) draft section 4).*

One key aspect of data governance is safeguarding the blinding of clinical trial data. The design and implementation of systems, user accounts, and delegation of responsibilities must keep the importance of protecting the blind in mind. All aspects of blinding should be documented with roles, responsibilities, and procedures where needed. To account for potential unblinding, the risk assessment should include a strategy for documenting and assessing the impact unblinding may have.

DATA LIFE CYCLE ELEMENTS

This section details the expanded requirement of procedures that should be in place to cover the full data life cycle, including data capture, relevant metadata (including audit trails), review of data and metadata, data corrections, data transfer, exchange, and migration, and the finalization of data sets prior to analysis.

Computerized Systems

This section further describes the need for the responsibilities of the sponsor, investigator, and other parties in terms of computerized systems used in clinical trials to be documented. It is important to note that with ICH E6(R3), computer systems are no longer solely the responsibility of the sponsor – they are now a responsibility shared among the sponsor, investigator, and involved parties.

Sponsors retain overall responsibility for ensuring computer systems used in a trial meet expectations and are risk-proportionate. For systems used by the investigator, the sponsor still has the responsibility to assess the systems to ensure they are fit for purpose for the trial. Investigator/institutionally deployed systems for trial conduct have the responsibility of meeting expectations and implementing them. Entities developing computerized systems for clinical trial use must be aware of the intended purpose and regulatory requirements applicable to the systems. For all systems used in clinical trials, documented procedures for appropriate use for the trial should be in place, and users should receive appropriate training prior to accessing and using these systems.

Security of Computerized Systems, Validation of Computerized Systems, System Failure, Technical Support

These four new sections under Computerized Systems in many ways mirror and expand on the requirements already covered by 21CFR11 (see Chapter 11). Tantamount is the protection and security of clinical trial data and records – these should be managed appropriately throughout the clinical trial lifecycle, including system validation, security measures, data backup, and disaster recovery, as required.

User Management

Any system utilized in a clinical trial must have appropriate access controls designed to limit access to only authorized users, such that all data can be attributed to an individual. User access must align with the user's role defined in the trial and must maintain data confidentiality and blinding. Documentation of all user access privileges should be maintained.

GLOSSARY

The glossary in ICH E6(R3) is moved to later in the guidance, and this revision brings some new and updated terms. Of note, trial subjects are now participants, and terms such as Computerized Systems, Validation, Data Acquisition Tool, Metadata, Reference Safety Information, Service Provider, and Signature are added. There are updated definitions for other terms that change how sponsors and investigators think about trial design and execution. The most significant change is Essential Documents, which are now called Essential Records and are discussed in greater detail below.

APPENDIX A: INVESTIGATOR'S BROCHURE

There are currently few proposed changes to the Investigator's Brochure from ICH E6(R2) to (R3), other than the placement of this section now as an appendix rather than in the body of the guidance.

APPENDIX B: CLINICAL TRIAL PROTOCOL AND PROTOCOL AMENDMENT(S)

Clinical trial protocols should describe the trial in a clear, concise, and operationally feasible manner that minimizes unnecessary complexity and risks. It should focus on the safety, rights, and well-being of the trial participant while generating reliable data. One additional requirement is that protocols should clearly address the implications for the withdrawal of informed consent from trial participants or the discontinuation by the investigator. ICH E6(R3) also highlights the need to build adaptability into protocols. This can be achieved by building acceptable ranges for specific protocol provisions, which can reduce the number of deviations or, in some cases, the need for a protocol amendment. There is also a focus on better integrating ICH E8(R1) and ICH E9 into the clinical trial protocol/amendments.

Additional considerations in this revision regarding protocols include streamlining many of the name and address requirements, including mechanisms for pre-screening and screening of trial participants and references to IDMCs or adjudication committees for safety and efficacy, as appropriate. The revision also updated the statistical considerations section to better align it with current practices. Quality assurance and quality control activities related to the trial were added and defined for inclusion in protocols. There is also now a section on data handling and record-keeping, ensuring alignment of expectations throughout and after the trial.

APPENDIX C: ESSENTIAL RECORDS FOR THE CONDUCT OF A CLINICAL TRIAL

This section, replacing ICH E6(R2) Section 8, represents a complete revision to the thinking of records versus documents and what is essential. To embrace the flexibility of clinical trial design, the guidance recognizes that what is essential may differ from trial to trial. To make the guidance proportionate to the needs of the trial, this section has been fully reworked to move away from a 'checklist' kind of thinking and put the responsibility of deciding what is essential for a given trial on the sponsor. The revision also moves away from separating records by trial stage (before the trial, during the conduct of the trial, and after completion of the trial) and instead recognizes the essentiality of records throughout a trial.

Records are now divided into two groups: those that are essential records for all trials and those that are potentially essential records. The guidance now provides a definition of the essentiality of trial records, along with criteria for determining whether a given record is essential for that trial. It is up to the sponsor to determine where the essential records are located (sponsor TMF or the investigator site file (ISF)); this is no longer pre-determined by the guidance.

This revised guidance also expands this section to provide more clarity on what is required and when, noting that the timeliness of records available in either the TMF or ISF is important to the successful management of the trial. Determining who needs access to records is a component of the essentiality of the records. The goal of this revision is to foster forward thinking from the sponsor and investigator on the records that may be needed to reconstruct the trial, if required at a future date.

CONCLUSION

This chapter highlights the most significant changes being considered in the modernization of ICH E6(R2). While there are many minor changes that were not discussed and may yet change – the major revisions discussed here provide insights into the fundamental revisions in the works to foster clinical trials that are of high quality, that identify and adequately manage and minimize risks, that address and manage the data lifecycle, all while focusing on the rights, safety, and well-being of trial participants.

For the current thinking and progress toward making ICH E6(R3) draft guidance effective, see the current draft ICH E6(R3) guidance,[1] the Expert Working Group Public Web Conference Report,[2] and a comparison of the E6(R2) to E6(R3) changes outlined in the Clinical Pathways tool for ICH E6(R3) vs. ICH E6(R2) comparison tool.[3]

NOTES

1 https://database.ich.org/sites/default/files/ICH_E6%28R3%29_DraftGuideline_2023_0519.pdf
2 https://database.ich.org/sites/default/files/ICH_E6R3_WebConference_Report_Final_2021_1011.pdf
3 https://www.clinicalpathwaysresearch.com/store/iche6r3-tool

5 Good Clinical Safety Practice

Karen Truhe

INTRODUCTION

For sponsors to take appropriate action with important safety information that arises during clinical development, there must be an understanding of common definitions and procedures to ensure Good Clinical Practice (GCP) in the area of safety and pharmacovigilance (PV).

Commonly used PV terms and their associated acronyms have evolved over the years and have been a source of confusion for clinical research professionals. The term 'pharmacovigilance' itself, defined by the World Health Organization (WHO) as "the science and activities relating to the detection, assessment, understanding and prevention of adverse effects or any other medicine/vaccine related problem,"[1] replaced the older 'drug safety' only within the last two decades.

In 1994, the International Conference on Harmonisation of Technical Requirements for Registration of Pharmaceuticals for Human Use (ICH) E2A guidance provided the industry with standard definitions and instructions on how to handle expedited reporting during the pre-approval phase. ICH E2A was adopted by the US Food and Drug Administration (FDA) and published in the Federal Register on March 1, 1995 and has been adopted in most countries.

In 2011, FDA's 2010 Final Rule became effective, with the goal of improving the quality of expedited safety reports received from clinical trials. The Final Rule also sought to eliminate terminology known to cause confusion and clarify the obligations of both the study sponsor and participating investigators. To facilitate the implementation of these regulatory changes, the FDA has developed several safety guidance documents to provide further recommendations.

Various guidance documents and other resources from regulators and working groups have been developed to inform the various stakeholders about their safety reporting responsibilities, yet confusion persists, leading to noncompliance, inspection findings and most importantly, risks to patient safety.

The concepts and recommendations in this chapter are intended to provide guidance for assessing and reporting safety information to minimize risks to subjects participating in clinical trials and to assist sponsors with GCP inspection readiness. They are also meant to ensure that the safety information collected during the pre-market phase aids in the development of a clinically meaningful benefit risk assessment as sponsors prepare marketing authorization applications.

DOI: 10.1201/9781003407010-5

DEFINITIONS AND TERMINOLOGY IN CLINICAL SAFETY

Before outlining expedited reporting requirements for adverse events that occur in the clinical trial setting, an understanding of common terms used in safety and PV is essential. The following definitions of these terms as they appear verbatim in E2A[2] are presented below in italicized text. The definitions are followed directly by comments and notes for interpretation.

Adverse Event

Any untoward medical occurrence in a patient or clinical investigation subject administered a pharmaceutical product and which does not necessarily have to have a causal relationship with this treatment.

An adverse event (AE) is "any unfavorable sign, symptom or outcome"[2] that occurs during the use of the drug (or placebo or active comparator) without implying the AE is related to the use of the drug.

The term 'causal relationship' used in the definition above will be referred to frequently throughout this chapter, so it is important to understand the concept. Put simply, the investigator and the sponsor must decide whether the drug caused the AE to occur or not. There have been multiple scales and systems developed to aid the clinical trial investigator and study sponsor in their determination of causal relationships. The CIOMS VI Working Group[3] recommends that investigators provide a simple binary "yes/no" (e.g., related, not related) causality assessment for adverse events.

Adverse Drug Reaction

In the pre-approval clinical experience with a new medicinal product or its new usages, particularly as the therapeutic dose(s) may not be established: all noxious and unintended responses to a medicinal product related to any dose should be considered adverse drug reactions.

The term adverse drug reaction (also referred to as adverse reaction) implies that the relationship between the drug and the adverse event (e.g., the causal relationship) is at least a "reasonable possibility."[2]

For the purposes of IND safety reporting, the FDA's interpretation of "reasonable possibility" means there is evidence to suggest a causal relationship between the drug and the adverse event (21 CFR 312.32(a)).[4]

Examples of reasonable possibilities provided in 21 CFR 312.32(c)(1)(i)[4] include:

- A single occurrence of an event that is uncommon and known to be strongly associated with drug exposure (e.g., angioedema, hepatic injury, Stevens-Johnson syndrome)
- One or more occurrences of an event that is not commonly associated with drug exposure but is otherwise uncommon in the population exposed to the drug (e.g., tendon rupture)

Unexpected Adverse Drug Reaction

An adverse reaction, the nature or severity of which is not consistent with the applicable product information (e.g., Investigator's Brochure for an unapproved investigational medicinal product).

It is worth noting that the terms "expected" and "unexpected" carry various interpretations within the field of medicine and are another common point of confusion when assessing adverse event reports. For the purposes of safety reporting, "expected" does not refer to what might be anticipated clinically in a certain patient population or within a drug class. Instead, "expected" should be interpreted as what is expected to occur with a particular drug under study as evidenced by what is listed in the Reference Safety Information (RSI) section of a product's Investigator's Brochure (IB). The expectedness assessment will ultimately determine if SAEs need to be reported to regulators in an expedited (rapid) or periodic manner.

The definition of unexpected in 21 CFR 312.32(a)[4] goes on to further state that an adverse event is considered unexpected if it is not listed in the IB or at the *specificity or severity* that has been observed with the drug under investigation. For example, if the IB refers only to 'anemia' as an expected serious adverse reaction (SAR) with the study drug, a report of 'hemolytic anemia' would be considered unexpected given the greater specificity.

In addition to these basic terms, sponsors conducting clinical research must also understand what meets the criteria for classification as a serious adverse event.

Per E2A,[2] an adverse event is considered serious if, at any dose, it:

- *Results in death*
- *Is life-threatening (Note: the term "life-threatening" in the definition of "serious" refers to an event in which the patient was at risk of death at the time of the event; it does not refer to an event that hypothetically might have caused death if it had been more severe.)*
- *Requires inpatient hospitalization or prolongation of existing hospitalization*
- *Results in a persistent or significant disability/incapacity*
- *Is a congenital anomaly/birth defect*
- *Is an important medical event that may not be immediately life-threatening or result in death or hospitalization but may jeopardize the patient or may require intervention to prevent one of the outcomes listed above. Examples of such events are intensive treatment in an emergency room or at home for allergic bronchospasm; blood dyscrasias or convulsions that do not result in hospitalization; or the development of drug dependency or drug abuse.*

A much more detailed list of potential important medical events was developed by the EudraVigilance Expert Working Group, along with a rationale for the inclusion/exclusion criteria used during the list's development.[5] This is a valuable resource for sponsors to consult during protocol development, as there may be important medical events specific to a patient population or drug that can be provided as examples when writing a protocol. The list is updated each time a new MedDRA version is released.

Seriousness should not be confused with the severity of an adverse event, which is another term mentioned throughout E2A.[2] Severity is used to describe the intensity of an adverse event (e.g., mild, moderate, or severe vomiting), while seriousness is associated with an outcome. Seriousness is a key element that drives the timeframe in which adverse events become reportable to health authorities, while severity is not.

WHICH CASES ARE SUBJECT TO EXPEDITED REPORTING?

Certain situations call for rapid reporting, so that all relevant stakeholders are made aware of new and important information that may impact patient safety.

The sponsor is required, per 21 CFR 312.32(c),[4] to notify the FDA and investigators through an IND safety report of the following potential serious risks. Examples can be found in 21 CFR 312.32(c)(i)[4] and additional detailed information in the FDA guidance documents on Safety Reporting Requirements for INDs and Bioavailability/Bioequivalence Studies.[6,7]

- **Serious Unexpected Suspected Adverse Reactions (SUSARs)** – cases that are serious, unexpected and for which there is evidence of a causal relationship between the drug and the AE. If all three criteria are not met, the case should not be submitted.
- **Other Observations** – the sponsor must also report on an expedited basis any findings that could suggest a significant risk to patients, change the benefit-risk profile of a product, require changes to study drug administration, or study conduct in general.
- Other observations defined in E2A[2] include, but are not limited to:
  a *An increase in the rate of occurrence, which is judged to be clinically important*
  b *A significant hazard to the patient population, such as a lack of efficacy with a medicinal product used in treating life-threatening disease.*
  c *A major safety finding from a newly completed animal study (such as carcinogenicity)*

WHEN TO REPORT

A case must include the following minimum criteria:

- an identifiable patient
- a suspect medicinal product
- an identifiable reporting source
- and an event or outcome that can be identified as unexpected

Once the sponsor obtains these minimum criteria (also known as the four elements of a case), the reporting clock begins. This is referred to as the "awareness date" or "Day 0."

- 7-Day IND Safety Reports
- Certain reports may contain important safety information on unexpected *fatal or life-threatening* adverse reactions occurring in clinical trials that require more rapid notification. Regulatory agencies require notification of these reports "as soon as possible," but no later than 7 calendar days after the sponsor first becomes aware of the event (e.g., the awareness date). The initial report need not be complete at this stage, but a follow-up with the complete information should be reported within 8 additional calendar days.
- 15-Day IND Safety Reports
- Reports that are not fatal or life-threatening but meet other seriousness and expedited reporting criteria must be reported as soon as possible, but no later than 15 calendar days after the sponsor first becomes aware of the event.

In most circumstances, SAEs will not be reported after a study's clinical conduct has concluded. However, if at any time an investigator becomes aware of important safety information on a study subject (typically one thought to be related to the use of the study drug), the event should be reported to the sponsor for evaluation and assessment.

HOW TO REPORT

The CIOMS I Form and FDA Form 3500 A are standard forms used for expedited safety reporting. Though paper-based reporting is still in practice, many agencies require reporting in an electronic format. This is constantly evolving, and sponsors must stay up to date on legislation and guidance in every country in which clinical trials are being conducted to ensure compliance.

The FDA recommends that sponsors submit IND Safety Reports in Electronic Common Technical Document (eCTD) format. Further details can be found in FDA Safety Reporting Guidance[6,7] and in 21 CFR 312.32.[4]

Prior to expedited reporting, it is recommended that the sponsor unblind the specific patient to determine whether or not the case truly meets the criteria for an expedited report (e.g., the ADR is actually unexpected for the study drug given to the subject).

It is also recommended that medical and biometrics personnel who will be responsible for end-of-study analysis and assessments remain blinded for the duration of the study. Sponsors may appoint an unblinded safety designee within the company or a third party to ensure good clinical practice and maintain the integrity of study blinding.

If, after unblinding, it is determined that a SUSAR is associated with an active comparator used in the study, the sponsor must decide whether these cases should be reported to the other manufacturer or directly to applicable health authorities.

In a study conducted under an IND, FDA guidance[6] recommends that sponsors notify the NDA or BLA holder of a marketed comparator product so that they can perform the necessary safety submissions.

In addition to regulators, investigators, and Institutional Review Boards (IRBs)/Ethics Committees (ECs) should be aware of new and significant safety information needed to protect study subjects.

To ensure investigators are aware of new and significant safety information needed to protect patients, the IB should be updated and provided to all active clinical trial sites in a timely manner.

CROSS-REPORTING OF SUSARS

A common question from sponsors is whether or not events occurring with one dosage form or indication that qualify for expedited reporting should be cross-reported to other INDs (or NDA/BLA, if applicable). While there is a chance that potential over-reporting could occur, E2A[2] recommends cross-reporting when qualifying reports are received for the same active moiety. Further information on cross reporting requirements for studies conducted under a US IND can be found in 21 CFR 312.32(c)(1)(ii)[4] and 312.32(c)(4).[4]

EXAMPLES OF INSPECTION FINDINGS

Examples of areas of concern related to safety and PV that were identified as findings during inspections by the Medicines and Healthcare Products Regulatory Agency (MHRA) GCP Inspectorate[8] are provided below. These examples could be useful to help sponsors address similar issues and prepare for GCP inspections.

- A critical finding for a pharmaceutical company identified the following issues:
    - "The format, implementation, and use of the RSI for expectedness assessments for serious Adverse Events (SAEs) and Serious Adverse Reactions (SARs) were not in accordance with CT-3 Guidance[9] and CTFG Q&A RSI (November 2017).[10] Therefore, there was significant potential for under-reporting of Suspected Unexpected Serious Adverse Reactions (SUSARs) due to the use of unapproved terms being classified as 'expected' events."
    - "There were more adverse reaction terms considered expected in the safety database used for SAR case assessment than contained in the RSI that had been approved by the MHRA in the Clinical Trial Authorisation (CTA)."
- A critical finding for a pharmaceutical company resulted after a review of corrective and preventive actions (CAPAs) from previous inspections was found to be ineffective.
    - "A number of events had been reported late as SUSARs due to an incorrect expectedness assessment upon the event becoming Fatal/Life Threatening. This demonstrated that the RSI was not being applied correctly to all cases upon initial receipt."
- A critical finding for a pharmaceutical company identified the following issues:

- "It was standard practice to assess 'lack of efficacy' events as 'expected', irrelevant of the terms that were listed in the approved RSI."
- "Examples were seen of SAEs being grouped as single cases in the safety database without adequate justification. For example, a second event of sepsis had been classified as a follow-up to an initial event of Sepsis and urinary tract infection under Neutropenic Sepsis."

- A critical finding for a pharmaceutical company resulted after a non-compliance from a prior inspection had not been addressed, and the company was still underreporting SUSARs.
  - "The process for updating, management, and implementation of the RSI remained undefined in the Standard Operating Procedures (SOPs)/Quality System."
  - "A number of discrepancies were identified in the safety database, which could have led to underreporting of SUSARs. For example, fatal events being classified as expected and disease progression/lack of efficacy/general health deterioration being classified as expected."

REFERENCES

1. World Health Organization (2023, May 2). Pharmacovigilance. https://www.who.int/teams/regulation-prequalification/regulation-and-safety/pharmacovigilance. Accessed November 19, 2023.
2. FDA Guidance for Industry (March 1995). E2A Clinical Safety Data Management: Definitions and Standards for Expedited Reporting.
3. Report of the Council for International Organizations of Medical Sciences (CIOMS) Working Group VI, 2005, Management of Safety Information from Clinical Trials. Report of CIOMS Working Group VI.
4. U.S. Food and Drug Administration (2011). Code of Federal Regulations Title 21 Food and Drugs Chapter I Food and Drug Administration Department of Health and Human Services Subchapter D Drugs for Human Use Part 312 Investigational New Drug Application.
5. Inclusion/Exclusion Criteria for the "Important Medical Events" List. European Medicines Agency. Published 18 March 2021. Available at https://www.ema.europa.eu/en/documents/other/inclusion-exclusion-criteria-important-medical-events-list-meddra_en.pdf. Accessed November 18, 2023.
6. FDA Guidance for Industry and Investigators (December 2012). Safety Reporting Requirements for INDs and BA/BE Studies.
7. FDA Draft Guidance for Industry (June 2021). Sponsor Responsibilities - Safety Reporting Requirements and Safety Assessment for IND and Bioavailability/Bioequivalence Studies.
8. MHRA. GCP Inspectorate. GCP Inspections Metrics Report. Metrics Period: 1st April 2019 to 31st March 2020 Report date: 29 March 2023 (re-issued 11 April 2023). Available at https://assets.publishing.service.gov.uk/government/uploads/system/uploads/attachment_data/file/1149658/GCP_inspection_metrics_2019-2020.pdf. Accessed November 19, 2023.
9. Information from European Union Institutions, Bodies, Offices and Agencies (EC): Communication from the Commission-Detailed Guidance on the Collection, Verification and Presentation of Adverse Event/Reaction Reports Arising from Clinical Trials. Official Journal of the European Union 2011;C 172/1.

10. Clinical Trial Facilitation Group (CTFG) (November 2017). Q&A Document-Reference Safety Information. Available at https://www.hma.eu/fileadmin/dateien/Human_Medicines/01-About_HMA/Working_Groups/CTFG/2017_11_CTFG_Question_and_Answer_on_Reference_Safety_Information_2017.pdf. Accessed November 19, 2023.

6 Informed Consent

Joseph Near

INTRODUCTION

Informed consent is an integral feature of the ethical conduct of a trial. Clinical trial participation should be voluntary and based on a consent process that ensures participants are well-informed.

Freely given informed consent should be obtained and documented from every participant prior to clinical trial participation.[1] For participants unable to provide informed consent, their legally authorized representative should provide consent prior to clinical trial participation.

The process and information provided should be designed to achieve the primary objective of enabling trial participants to make an informed decision on whether or not to participate in the trial.[1] The informed consent process should take into consideration relevant aspects of the trial, such as the characteristics of the participants, the trial design, the anticipated benefit and risk of medical intervention(s), the setting and context in which the trial will be conducted (e.g., trials in emergency situations), and the potential use of technology to inform participants and obtain informed consent.

The regulatory requirements for obtaining informed consent to participate in clinical trials are delineated in 21 Code of Federal Regulations (CFR) Part 50 – Protection of Human Subjects, Subparts A (General Provisions), B (Informed Consent of Human Subjects), and D (Additional Safeguards for Children in Clinical Investigations); and in Section 4.8 (Informed Consent of Trial Subjects) of ICH GCP E6(R2) Good Clinical Practice, Guidance for Industry.

REGULATIONS

21 CFR Part 50 Subpart A (Protection of Subjects, General Provisions)

This section defines the scope of activities to which this provision of the regulations applies, including:

All clinical investigations regulated by the Food and Drug Administration under sections 505(i) and 520(g) of the Federal Food, Drug, and Cosmetic Act, as well as clinical investigations that support applications for research or marketing permits for products regulated by the Food and Drug Administration, including foods, dietary supplements that bear a nutrient content claim or a health claim, infant formulas, food and color additives, drugs for human use, medical devices for human use, biological products for human use, and electronic products. Additional specific obligations and commitments of, and standards of conduct for, persons who sponsor or monitor clinical investigations involving particular test articles may also be found in other parts (e.g., parts 312 and 812).[2] *Compliance with these parts is*

DOI: 10.1201/9781003407010-6

intended to protect the rights and safety of subjects involved in investigations filed with the Food and Drug Administration pursuant to sections 403, 406, 409, 412, 413, 502, 503, 505, 510, 513–516, 518–520, 721, and 801 of the Federal Food, Drug, and Cosmetic Act and sections 351 and 354–360F of the Public Health Service Act.

This section also provides definitions of terms used in the regulation.

21 CFR Part 50 Subpart B (Protection of Subjects, Informed Consent of Human Subjects)

This section explains the general requirements for informed consent as well as exceptions from the general requirements and states:

Except as provided in the Exceptions from the General Requirements, no investigator may involve a human being as a subject in research covered by these regulations unless the investigator has obtained the legally effective informed consent of the subject or the subject's legally authorized representative. An investigator shall seek such consent only under circumstances that provide the prospective subject or the representative with sufficient opportunity to consider whether or not to participate and that minimize the possibility of coercion or undue influence. The information that is given to the subject or the representative shall be in language understandable to the subject or the representative. No informed consent, whether oral or written, may include any exculpatory language through which the subject or the representative is made to waive or appear to waive any of the subject's legal rights, or releases or appears to release the investigator, the sponsor, the institution, or its agents from liability for negligence.

Under the *Exceptions from the General Requirements* section, the regulations state that obtaining informed consent shall be deemed feasible unless, before use of the test article, both the investigator and a physician who is not otherwise participating in the clinical investigation certify in writing all of the following:

1. The human subject is confronted by a life-threatening situation necessitating the use of the test article.
2. Informed consent cannot be obtained from the subject due to an inability to communicate with, or obtain legally effective consent from, the subject.
3. Time is not sufficient to obtain consent from the subject's legal representative.
4. No alternative method of approved or generally recognized therapy is available that provides an equal or greater likelihood of saving the life of the subject.

If immediate use of the test article is, in the investigator's opinion, required to preserve the life of the subject and time is not sufficient to obtain the independent determination in advance of using the test article, the determinations of the clinical investigator shall be made and, within five working days after the use of the article, reviewed and evaluated in writing by a physician who is not participating in the clinical investigation, and the required documentation shall be submitted to the Institutional Review Board (IRB) within five working days after the use of the test article.

This is followed by a section that details the presidential waiver of the prior consent requirements for the administration of an investigational new drug to a member of the armed forces in connection with the member's participation in a particular military operation as defined in 10 U.S.C. 1107(f) and exceptions from informed consent requirements for emergency research.

Elements of Informed Consent

This section details the basic elements of informed consent that shall be provided to each subject and includes:

1. *A statement that the study involves research, an explanation of the purposes of the research and the expected duration of the subject's participation, a description of the procedures to be followed, and identification of any procedures that are experimental.*
2. *A description of any reasonably foreseeable risks or discomforts to the subject.*
3. *A description of any benefits to the subject or to others that may reasonably be expected from the research.*
4. *A disclosure of appropriate alternative procedures or courses of treatment, if any, that might be advantageous to the subject.*
5. *A statement describing the extent, if any, to which confidentiality of records identifying the subject will be maintained and that notes the possibility that the Food and Drug Administration may inspect the records.*
6. *For research involving more than minimal risk, an explanation as to whether any compensation and an explanation as to whether any medical treatments are available if injury occurs, and, if so, what they consist of, or where further information may be obtained.*
7. *An explanation of whom to contact for answers to pertinent questions about the research and research subjects' rights, and whom to contact in the event of a research-related injury to the subject.*
8. *A statement that participation is voluntary, that refusal to participate will involve no penalty or loss of benefits to which the subject is otherwise entitled, and that the subject may discontinue participation at any time without penalty or loss of benefits to which the subject is otherwise entitled.*

Additional Elements of Informed Consent

This section details information that shall also be provided to each subject when appropriate and includes:

1. *A statement that the particular treatment or procedure may involve risks to the subject (or to the embryo or fetus, if the subject is or may become pregnant), which are currently unforeseeable.*
2. *Anticipated circumstances under which the subject's participation may be terminated by the investigator without regard to the subject's consent.*
3. *Any additional costs to the subject that may result from participation in the research.*
4. *The consequences of a subject's decision to withdraw from the research and procedures for orderly termination of participation by the subject.*

5. *A statement stating that significant new findings developed during the course of the research that may relate to the subject's willingness to continue participation will be provided to the subject.*
6. *The approximate number of subjects involved in the study.*

Clinical Trial Registry Databank (ct.gov)

The regulations also require that when seeking informed consent for applicable clinical trials, as defined in 42 U.S.C. 282(j)(1)(A), the following statement shall be provided to each clinical trial subject in informed consent documents and processes. This will notify the clinical trial subject that clinical trial information has been or will be submitted for inclusion in the clinical trial registry databank under paragraph (j) of section 402 of the Public Health Service Act. The statement is: "A description of this clinical trial will be available on *http://www.ClinicalTrials.gov*, as required by U.S. Law. This web site will not include information that can identify you. At most, the web site will include a summary of the results. You can search this Web site at any time."

Documentation of Informed Consent

This section indicates that informed consent shall be documented by the use of a written consent form approved by the IRB and signed and dated by the subject or the subject's legally authorized representative at the time of consent, and a copy shall be given to the person signing the form. The consent form may be either of the following:

1. A written consent document that embodies the elements of informed consent. This form may be read to the subject or the subject's legally authorized representative, but, in any event, the investigator shall give either the subject or the representative adequate opportunity to read it before it is signed.
2. A *short-form* written consent document stating that the required elements of informed consent have been presented orally to the subject or the subject's legally authorized representative. When this method is used, there shall be a witness to the oral presentation. Also, the IRB shall approve a written summary of what is to be said to the subject or the representative. Only the short form itself is to be signed by the subject or the representative. However, the witness shall sign both the short form and a copy of the summary, and the person actually obtaining the consent shall sign a copy of the summary. A copy of the summary shall be given to the subject or the representative in addition to a copy of the *short form.*

21 CFR Part 50 Subpart D (Additional Safeguards for Children in Clinical Investigations)

IRB Duties

In addition to other responsibilities assigned to IRBs under these regulations, each IRB must review clinical investigations involving children as subjects and approve only those clinical investigations that satisfy the criteria described below and the conditions of all other applicable elements of 21 CFR Part 50.

Clinical Investigations Not Involving Greater Than Minimal Risk

Any clinical investigation within the scope of 21 CFR Part 50 in which no greater than minimal risk to children is presented may involve children as subjects only if the IRB finds that:

1. *No greater than minimal risk to children is presented; and*
2. *Adequate provisions are made for soliciting the assent of the children and the permission of their parents or guardians.*

Clinical Investigations Involving Greater Than Minimal Risk but Presenting the Prospect of Direct Benefit to Individual Subjects

Any clinical investigation within the scope of 21 CFR Part 50 in which more than minimal risk to children is presented by an intervention or procedure that holds out the prospect of direct benefit for the individual subject, or by a monitoring procedure that is likely to contribute to the subject's well-being, may involve children as subjects only if the IRB finds that:

1. *The risk is justified by the anticipated benefit to the subjects;*
2. *The relation of the anticipated benefit to the risk is at least as favorable to the subjects as that presented by available alternative approaches; and*
3. *Adequate provisions are made for soliciting the assent of the children and the permission of their parents or guardians, as set forth in the applicable regulations.*

Clinical Investigations Involving Greater Than Minimal Risk and No Prospect of Direct Benefit to Individual Subjects, but Likely to Yield Generalizable Knowledge about the Subjects' Disorder or Condition

Any clinical investigation within the scope described in 21 CFR Part 50 in which more than minimal risk to children is presented by an intervention or procedure that does not hold out the prospect of direct benefit for the individual subject, or by a monitoring procedure that is not likely to contribute to the well-being of the subject, may involve children as subjects only if the IRB finds that:

1. *The risk represents a minor increase over a minimal risk;*
2. *The intervention or procedure presents experiences to subjects that are reasonably commensurate with those inherent in their actual or expected medical, dental, psychological, social, or educational situations;*
3. *The intervention or procedure is likely to yield generalizable knowledge about the subjects' disorder or condition that is of vital importance for the understanding or amelioration of the subjects' disorder or condition; and*
4. *Adequate provisions are made for soliciting the assent of the children and the permission of their parents or guardians, as set forth in the applicable section of the regulations.*

Clinical Investigations Not Otherwise Approvable that Present an Opportunity to Understand, Prevent, or Alleviate a Serious Problem Affecting the Health or Welfare of Children

If an IRB does not believe that a clinical investigation within the scope described in the applicable section of 21 CFR Part 50 and involving children as subjects meets the applicable requirements, the clinical investigation may proceed only if:

1. *The IRB finds that the clinical investigation presents a reasonable opportunity to further the understanding, prevention, or alleviation of a serious problem affecting the health or welfare of children; and*
2. *The Commissioner of Food and Drugs, after consultation with a panel of experts in pertinent disciplines (for example, science, medicine, education, ethics, and law) and following the opportunity for public review and comment, determines either:*
   a. *That the clinical investigation in fact satisfies the applicable conditions of 21 CFR Part 50, or*
   b. *The following conditions are met:*
      i. *The clinical investigation presents a reasonable opportunity to further the understanding, prevention, or alleviation of a serious problem affecting the health or welfare of children;*
      ii. *The clinical investigation will be conducted in accordance with sound ethical principles; and*
      iii. *Adequate provisions are made for soliciting the assent of children and the permission of their parents or guardians, as set forth in the applicable section of the regulations.*

Requirements for Permission by Parents or Guardians and for Assent by Children

In addition to the determinations required under other applicable sections of this subpart D, the IRB must determine that adequate provisions are made for soliciting the assent of the children when, in the judgment of the IRB, the children are capable of providing assent.

In determining whether children are capable of providing assent, the IRB must take into account the ages, maturity, and psychological state of the children involved. This judgment may be made for all children to be involved in clinical investigations under a particular protocol or for each child, as the IRB deems appropriate.

The assent of the children is not a necessary condition for proceeding with the clinical investigation if the IRB determines:

1. That the capability of some or all of the children is so limited that they cannot reasonably be consulted, or
2. That the intervention or procedure involved in the clinical investigation holds out a prospect of direct benefit that is important to the health or well-being of the children and is available only in the context of the clinical investigation.

Even where the IRB determines that the subjects are capable of assenting, the IRB may still waive the assent requirement if it finds and documents that:

1. The clinical investigation involves no more than minimal risk to the subjects. The waiver will not adversely affect the rights and welfare of the subjects;
2. The clinical investigation could not practicably be carried out without the waiver; and
3. Whenever appropriate, the subjects will be provided with additional pertinent information after participation.

In addition to the determinations required under other applicable sections of this subpart D, the IRB must determine, in accordance with and to the extent that consent is required under 21 CFR Part 50, that the permission of each child's parents or guardian is granted.

1. *Where parental permission is to be obtained, the IRB may find that the permission of one parent is sufficient for clinical investigations.*
2. *Where clinical investigations are covered by the applicable sections of 21 CFR Part 50 and permission is to be obtained from parents, both parents must give their permission unless one parent is deceased, unknown, incompetent, or not reasonably available, or when only one parent has legal responsibility for the care and custody of the child.*

Permission by parents or guardians must be documented in accordance with and to the extent required by the applicable sections of 21 CFR Part 50.

When the IRB determines that assent is required, it must also determine whether and how assent must be documented.

Wards

Children who are wards of the state or any other agency, institution, or entity can be included in clinical investigations approved under 21 CFR Part 50 only if such clinical investigations are:

1. *Related to their status as wards; or*
2. *Conducted in schools, camps, hospitals, institutions, or similar settings in which the majority of children involved as subjects are not wards*

If the clinical investigation is approved under the above section, the IRB must require the appointment of an advocate for each child who is a ward.

1. The advocate will serve in addition to any other individual acting on behalf of the child as guardian or in loco parentis.
2. One individual may serve as an advocate for more than one child.

3. The advocate must be an individual who has the background and experience to act in, and agrees to act in, the best interest of the child for the duration of the child's participation in the clinical investigation.
4. The advocate must not be associated in any way (except in the role of advocate or member of the IRB) with the clinical investigation, the investigator(s), or the guardian organization.

ICH GCP E6(R2) Good Clinical Practice, Guidance for Industry, Section 4.8, Informed Consent of Trial Subjects

ICH GCP E6(R2) delineates elements of the informed consent process including how informed consent is to be obtained, the language used in informed consent forms, and the content of informed consent forms. Specific requirements are provided below.

4.8.1 In obtaining and documenting informed consent, the investigator should comply with the applicable regulatory requirement(s) and adhere to GCP and the ethical principles that have their origin in the Declaration of Helsinki. Prior to the beginning of the trial, the investigator should have the IRB/IEC's written approval/favorable opinion of the written informed consent form and any other written information to be provided to subjects.

4.8.2 The written informed consent form and any other written information to be provided to subjects should be revised whenever important new information becomes available that may be relevant to the subject's consent. Any revised written informed consent form and written information should receive the IRB/IEC's approval/favorable opinion in advance of use. The subject or the subject's legally acceptable representative should be informed in a timely manner if new information becomes available that may be relevant to the subject's willingness to continue participation in the trial. The communication of this information should be documented.

4.8.3 Neither the investigator nor the trial staff should coerce or unduly influence a subject to participate or to continue to participate in a trial.

4.8.4 None of the oral and written information concerning the trial, including the written informed consent form, should contain any language that causes the subject or the subject's legally acceptable representative to waive or to appear to waive any legal rights, or that releases or appears to release the investigator, the institution, the sponsor, or their agents from liability for negligence.

4.8.5 The investigator, or a person designated by the investigator, should fully inform the subject or, if the subject is unable to provide informed consent, the subject's legally acceptable representative, of all pertinent aspects of the trial, including the written information and the approval/ favorable opinion by the IRB/IEC.

4.8.6 The language used in the oral and written information about the trial, including the written informed consent form, should be as non-technical as practical and should be understandable to the subject or the subject's legally acceptable representative and the impartial witness, where applicable.

4.8.7 Before informed consent may be obtained, the investigator, or a person designated by the investigator, should provide the subject or the subject's legally acceptable representative with ample time and opportunity to inquire about the details of the trial and to decide whether or not to participate in the trial. All questions about the trial should be answered to the satisfaction of the subject or the subject's legally acceptable representative.

4.8.8 Prior to a subject's participation in the trial, the written informed consent form should be signed and personally dated by the subject, by the subject's legally acceptable representative, and by the person who conducted the informed consent discussion.

4.8.9 If a subject is unable to read or if a legally acceptable representative is unable to read, an impartial witness should be present during the entire informed consent discussion. After the written informed consent form and any other written information to be provided to subjects is read and explained to the subject or the subject's legally acceptable representative, and after the subject or the subject's legally acceptable representative has orally consented to the subject's participation in the trial and, if capable of doing so, has signed and personally dated the informed consent form, the witness should sign and personally date the consent form. By signing the consent form, the witness attests that the information in the consent form and any other written information was accurately explained to, and apparently understood by, the subject or the subject's legally acceptable representative, and that informed consent was freely given by the subject or the subject's legally acceptable representative.

4.8.10 Both the informed consent discussion and the written informed consent form and any other written information to be provided to subjects should include explanations of the following:

a. That the trial involves research.
b. The purpose of the trial.
c. The trial treatment(s) and the probability for random assignment to each treatment.
d. The trial procedures to be followed, including all invasive procedures.
e. The subject's responsibilities.
f. Those aspects of the trial that are experimental.
g. The reasonably foreseeable risks or inconveniences to the subject and, when applicable, to an embryo, fetus, or nursing infant.
h. The reasonably expected benefits. When there is no intended clinical benefit to the subject, the subject should be made aware of this.
i. The alternative procedure(s) or course(s) of treatment that may be available to the subject and their important potential benefits and risks.
j. The compensation and/or treatment available to the subject in the event of a trial-related injury.
k. The anticipated prorated payment, if any, to the subject for participating in the trial.

l. The anticipated expenses, if any, to the subject for participating in the trial.
m. That the subject's participation in the trial is voluntary and that the subject may refuse to participate or withdraw from the trial, at any time, without penalty or loss of benefits to which the subject is otherwise entitled.
n. That the monitor(s), the auditor(s), the IRB/IEC, and the regulatory authority(ies) will be granted direct access to the subject's original medical records for verification of clinical trial procedures and/or data, without violating the confidentiality of the subject, to the extent permitted by the applicable laws and regulations, and that, by signing a written informed consent form, the subject or the subject's legally acceptable representative is authorizing such access.
o. That records identifying the subject will be kept confidential and, to the extent permitted by the applicable laws and/or regulations, will not be made publicly available. If the results of the trial are published, the subject's identity will remain confidential.
p. That the subject or the subject's legally acceptable representative will be informed in a timely manner if information becomes available that may be relevant to the subject's willingness to continue participation in the trial.
q. The person(s) to contact for further information regarding the trial and the rights of trial subjects, and whom to contact in the event of a trial-related injury.
r. The foreseeable circumstances and/or reasons under which the subject's participation in the trial may be terminated.
s. The expected duration of the subject's participation in the trial.
t. The approximate number of subjects involved in the trial.

4.8.11 Prior to participation in the trial, the subject or the subject's legally acceptable representative should receive a copy of the signed and dated written informed consent form and any other written information provided to the subject. During a subject's participation in the trial, the subject or the subject's legally acceptable representative should receive a copy of the signed and dated consent form updates and a copy of any amendments to the written information provided to subjects.

4.8.12 When a clinical trial (therapeutic or non-therapeutic) includes subjects who can only be enrolled in the trial with the consent of the subject's legally acceptable representative (e.g., minors, or patients with severe dementia), the subject should be informed about the trial to the extent compatible with the subject's understanding, and, if capable, the subject should sign and personally date the written informed consent.

4.8.13 Except as described in 4.8.14, a non-therapeutic trial (i.e., a trial in which there is no anticipated direct clinical benefit to the subject) should be conducted with subjects who personally give consent and who sign and date the written informed consent form.

4.8.14 Nontherapeutic trials may be conducted on subjects with the consent of a legally acceptable representative, provided the following conditions are fulfilled:

a. The objectives of the trial cannot be met by means of a trial with subjects who can give informed consent personally.
b. The foreseeable risks to the subjects are low.
c. The negative impact on the subject's well-being is minimized and low.
d. The trial is not prohibited by law.
e. The approval/favorable opinion of the IRB/IEC is expressly sought on the inclusion of such subjects, and the written approval/ favorable opinion covers this aspect.

Such trials, unless an exception is justified, should be conducted in patients with a disease or condition for which the investigational product is intended. Subjects in these trials should be particularly closely monitored and should be withdrawn if they appear to be unduly distressed.

4.8.15 In emergency situations where prior consent from the subject is not possible, the consent of the subject's legally acceptable representative, if present, should be requested. When prior consent of the subject is not possible and the subject's legally acceptable representative is not available, enrollment of the subject should require measures described in the protocol and/or elsewhere, with documented approval/favorable opinion by the IRB/IEC, to protect the rights, safety, and well-being of the subject and to ensure compliance with applicable regulatory requirements. The subject or the subject's legally acceptable representative should be informed about the trial as soon as possible, and consent to continue and other consent as appropriate (see Section 4.8.10) should be requested.

SPONSOR PROCESS FOR INFORMED CONSENT

Sponsors typically have a standard operating procedure (SOP) or similar controlled document describing how they manage informed consent forms, or they may rely upon a Contract Research Organization's (CROs) procedures for managing this process. The procedure should define roles and responsibilities for each element of the development and approval of informed consent forms (ICF), including the Trial-specific Master ICF, Supplemental ICFs, and Assent Forms.

Supplemental ICFs may be used to document informed consent for subject participation in an optional separate research study associated with a clinical trial, including storage and analysis of samples outside of clinical protocol requirements.

Assent forms are typically used for minor children or vulnerable subjects who are incapable of providing consent and must meet the requirements designated by the Institutional Review Board

(IRB)/Independent Ethics Committee (IEC) with oversight responsibilities for the clinical trial. Assent forms should be completed unless the child meets the requirements for verbal assent; however, the child's verbal assent should be documented, and the child's legal representative should sign the appropriate consent form.

The procedure should:

a. define the numbering system for ICFs, supplemental ICFs, and assent forms;
b. identify a system for tracking ICFs, supplemental ICFs, and assent forms;
c. ensure that ICF, supplemental ICFs, and assent form templates are updated when changes to the product Investigator's Brochure are made and ad hoc when changes to language regarding risks and benefits, injury, insurance, authorization language, birth control requirements, expenses and payments, confidentiality/data protection, and any other language that would be expected to be standardized across clinical trials are necessary,
d. ensure that the trial-specific templates are translated, with documented certificates, as necessary to support the population of the clinical trial,
e. ensure that revisions made to ICFs, supplemental ICFs, and assent forms meet specific country, and/or local IRB/IEC requirements are tracked.

The elements listed in ICH E6(R2) GCPs sections 4.8.10 a-t (see above) are an excellent basis upon which to create an ICF review and approval checklist.

INSPECTIONAL FINDINGS REGARDING INFORMED CONSENT

US FDA inspection findings related to ICFs tend to be most frequently identified at the site level. For example, the Fiscal Year (FY) 2022 Clinical Investigator FDA 483 observation trends identified the following ICF-related observations during inspections of clinical investigators.

Protocol Compliance Themes:

a. Revised informed consent not obtained or not obtained in a timely manner,
b. Informed consent not obtained prior to screening or investigational product administration,
c. Informed consent not obtained for a sub-study,
d. ICF copy not provided to subject,
e. ICF changes not approved by the IRB.

PREAMBLES

Each time the FDA develops rules to enact a law it provides the public an opportunity to comment on the agency's proposal, typically in the Federal Register (FR). Below are references to examples of "preambles" related to informed consent and may be of interest to individuals who want more information such as:

- Why the regulation is being proposed;
- The FDA's interpretation of the meaning and impact of the proposed regulation;
- The FDA's view and commentary on any comments received to the proposed rule;
  - Protection of Human Subjects; Informed Consent (January 27, 1981)

- Protection of Human Subjects; Clinical Investigations Which may be Reviewed Through Expedited Review Procedures Set Forth in FDA Regulations (January 27, 1981)
- Federal Policy for the Protection of Human Subjects (June 18, 1991)
- FDA Policy for the Protection of Human Subjects (June 18, 1991)
- Protection of Human Subjects; Informed Consent; Proposed Rule (September 21, 1995)
- Protection of Human Subjects; Informed Consent; Part II (October 2, 1996)
- Protection of Human Subjects; Informed Consent and Waiver of Informed Consent Requirements in Certain Emergency Research; Final Rule (October 2, 1996)
- Protection of Human Subjects; Informed Consent (December 22, 1995)
- Protection of Human Subjects; Informed Consent Verification; Final Rule (November 5, 1996)
- Protection of Human Subjects; Informed Consent; Exception from General Requirements (October 5, 1999)
- Additional Protection for Children (66 FR 20589-600) (April 24, 2001)
- Exception from General Requirements for Informed Consent (71 FR32827) (June 7, 2006)

REFERENCES

1 ICH-E6. Good Clinical Practice (GCP), Explanatory Note, 19 April 2021.
2 E6(R2). Good Clinical Practice: Integrated Addendum to ICH E6(R1) Guidance for Industry. U.S. Department of Health and Human Services, Food and Drug Administration, OMB Control No. 0910-0014.

7 Financial Disclosure by Clinical Investigators

Glenda Guest

Note that throughout this chapter, verbatim quotes from the Financial Disclosure Regulation, 21 CFR Part 54,[1] and FDA guidance entitled Financial Disclosure Guidance for Clinical Investigators, Industry and FDA Staff[2] are presented in italicized text, followed by additional comments and interpretation notes.

While each of the three main medical product centers at the FDA (the Center for Drug Evaluation and Research [CDER], the Center for Biologics Evaluation and Research [CBER], and the Center for Devices and Radiological Health [CDRH]) has slightly different missions with regard to the approval or clearance of medical products for the US market, they share the goal of ensuring the products are safe and effective. Assessment of potential bias is one key consideration in determining whether an application is approved under existing statutory requirements.

PURPOSE

a. *The Food and Drug Administration (FDA) evaluates clinical studies submitted in marketing applications, required by law, for new human drugs wand biological products and marketing applications and reclassification petitions for medical devices.*
b. *The agency reviews data generated in these clinical studies to determine whether the applications are approvable under the statutory requirements. FDA may consider clinical studies inadequate and the data inadequate if, among other things, appropriate steps have not been taken in the design, conduct, reporting, and analysis of the studies to minimize bias. One potential source of bias in clinical studies is a financial interest of the clinical investigator in the outcome of the study because of the way payment is arranged (e.g., a royalty) or because the investigator has a proprietary interest in the product (e.g., a patent) or because the investigator has an equity interest in the sponsor of the covered study. This section and conforming regulations require an applicant whose submission relies in part on clinical data to disclose certain financial arrangements between sponsor(s) of the covered studies and the clinical investigators and certain interests of the clinical investigators in the product under study or in the sponsor of the covered studies. FDA will use this information, in conjunction with*

DOI: 10.1201/9781003407010-7

information about the design and purpose of the study, as well as information obtained through on-site inspections, in the agency's assessment of the reliability of the data.[1]

FDA has justified implementation of the Financial Disclosure regulation by referencing *21 CFR Part 314.126 Adequate and Well-controlled Clinical Studies which stipulates (a) The purpose of conducting clinical investigations of a drug is to distinguish the effect of a drug from other influences, such as spontaneous change in the course of the disease, placebo effect,* ***or biased observation*** (emphasis added). *Reports of adequate and well-controlled investigations provide the primary basis for determining whether there is "substantial evidence" to support the claims of effectiveness for new drugs. Therefore, the study report should provide sufficient details of study design, conduct, and analysis to allow critical evaluation and a determination of whether the characteristics of an adequate and well-controlled study are present*[2].

While the above-quoted regulation[3] does not specifically refer to financial disclosure, it does refer to the underlying requirement to eliminate potential sources of bias in study conduct, analysis, and reporting.

Compliance with the requirements of the Financial Disclosure Regulation requires an understanding of the definitions and responsibilities for applicants, sponsors, clinical investigators, covered clinical studies, and the various types of financial arrangements that must be reported as well as the scope of the regulation.

DEFINITIONS

For the purposes of this part:

a. ***Compensation affected by the outcome of clinical studies*** *means compensation that could be higher for a favorable outcome than for an unfavorable outcome, such as compensation that is explicitly greater for a favorable result or compensation to the investigator in the form of an equity interest in the sponsor of a covered study or in the form of compensation tied to sales of the product, such as a royalty interest.*
b. ***Significant equity interest in the sponsor of a covered study*** *means any ownership interest, stock options, or other financial interest whose value cannot be readily determined through reference to public prices (generally, interests in a nonpublicly traded corporation), or any equity interest in a publicly traded corporation that exceeds $50,000 during the time the clinical investigator is carrying out the study and for 1 year following completion of the study.*
c. ***Proprietary interest in the tested product*** *means property or other financial interest in the product including, but not limited to, a patent, trademark, copyright or licensing agreement.*
d. ***Clinical investigator*** *means only a listed or identified investigator or subinvestigator who is directly involved in the treatment or evaluation of*

research subjects. The term also includes the spouse and each dependent child of the investigator.

e. ***Covered clinical study*** *means any study of a drug or device in humans submitted in a marketing application or reclassification petition subject to this part that the applicant or FDA relies on to establish that the product is effective (including studies that show equivalence to an effective product) or any study in which a single investigator makes a significant contribution to the demonstration of safety. This would, in general, not include phase l tolerance studies or pharmacokinetic studies, most clinical pharmacology studies (unless they are critical to an efficacy determination), large open safety studies conducted at multiple sites, treatment protocols, and parallel track protocols. An applicant may consult with FDA as to which clinical studies constitute "covered clinical studies" for purposes of complying with financial disclosure requirements.*

f. ***Significant payments of other sorts*** *mean payments made by the sponsor of a covered study to the investigator or the institution to support activities of the investigator that have a monetary value of more than $25,000, exclusive of the costs of conducting the clinical study or other clinical studies (e.g., a grant to fund ongoing research, compensation in the form of equipment or retainers for ongoing consultation or honoraria) during the time the clinical investigator is carrying out the study and for 1 year following the completion of the study.*

g. ***Applicant*** *means the party who submits a marketing application to FDA for approval of a drug, device, or biologic product. The applicant is responsible for submitting the appropriate certification and disclosure statements required in this part.*

h. ***Sponsor of the covered clinical study*** *means the party supporting a particular study at the time it was carried out.*[1]

It is important to understand that the reporting obligations include the spouse and dependent children of the clinical investigator and subinvestigator(s) during and for 1 year following completion of the study. Also, a clinical investigator would be required to report payments in excess of $25,000 made to an institution to support the activities of the clinical investigator.

While a definition of clinical investigator is provided within the regulation, one should be aware that the definition in 21 CFR Part 54 differs slightly between Parts 312 and 812 and the guidance document.

The guidance document offers this additional clarification (question D.1): *This definition is intended to identify the individuals for whom reporting under this regulation is required. Generally, these individuals are considered to be the investigators and subinvestigators taking responsibility for the study at a given study site. The definition also includes the spouse and each dependent child of such an investigator or subinvestigator. It should be noted that hospital staff, including nurses, residents, fellows, and office staff who provide ancillary or intermittent care but who do not make direct and significant contribution to the data are not meant to be included under the definition of clinical investigator. Additionally, individuals who only collect specimens or perform routine tests (such as blood pressure, EKG, x-ray) are not meant to be included under the definition of clinical investigator for purposes of financial disclosure.*[2]

SCOPE

The requirements in this part apply to any applicant who submits a marketing application for a human drug, biological product, or device and who submits covered clinical studies. The applicant is responsible for making the appropriate certification or disclosure statement where the applicant either contracted with one or more clinical investigators to conduct the studies or submitted studies conducted by others not under contract to the applicant.[1]

Note that the applicant and sponsor may not be the same entity, and that there may in fact be more than one sponsor for the clinical study.

The guidance document (question E.2) clarifies this as follows:

In many cases, the IND/IDE sponsor, the part 54 sponsor, and the applicant will be the same party. However, there may be times when they are not. For example, consider the case when an academic institution serves as the IND/IDE sponsor and a drug company serves as the part 54 sponsor by providing funding or the investigational drug for the study. When a marketing application is submitted, the drug company is likely to be the applicant. If, however, the drug company was sold to another company, the applicant may be neither the IND/IDE sponsor nor a part 54 sponsor.

It should be noted, however, that even if the IND/IDE sponsor will not be submitting the marketing application, the IND/IDE sponsor is still responsible for collecting financial information from the clinical investigators. The responsibility for reporting financial information to FDA falls upon the applicant; that is, part 54 requires the applicant to submit financial information when the marketing application is submitted to FDA.[2]

Compliance with the requirements of 21 CFR Part 54 requires a collaborative effort between sponsors and clinical investigators. To determine whether a disclosable financial interest exists, the sponsor must rely on the information provided by the clinical investigator. This includes the clinical investigator reporting the financial interests of specified family members and the requirement for self and family reporting by subinvestigators, as noted in the definition above.

Thus, understanding the roles of sponsor and applicant can at times be challenging. It is important that the shared obligations for financial disclosure be executed with diligence by the clinical investigators engaged in covered clinical studies, as well as sponsors, at the time the studies are conducted; otherwise, the applicant may bear additional burden in attempting to obtain the required information at the time an application is prepared for submission.

CERTIFICATION AND DISCLOSURE REQUIREMENTS

For purposes of this part, an applicant must submit a list of all clinical investigators who conducted covered clinical studies to determine whether the applicant's product meets the FDA's marketing requirements, identifying those clinical investigators who are full-time or part-time employees of the sponsor of each covered study. The applicant must also completely and accurately disclose or certify information concerning the financial interests of a clinical investigator who is not a full-time or part-time employee of the sponsor for each covered clinical study. Clinical investigators subject to investigational new drug or investigational device exemption regulations must provide the sponsor of the study with sufficient accurate information needed to allow subsequent disclosure or certification. The applicant is required to submit for each clinical investigator who participates in a covered study either a certification that none of the financial arrangements described in 54.2 exist, or disclose the nature of those arrangements to the agency. Where the applicant acts with due diligence to obtain the information required in this section but is unable to do so, the applicant shall certify that despite the applicant's due diligence in attempting to obtain the information, the applicant was unable to obtain the information and shall include the reason.

a. *The applicant (of an application submitted under sections 505, 506, 510(k), 513, or 515 of the Federal Food, Drug, and Cosmetic Act, or section 351 of the Public Health Service Act) that relies in whole or in part on clinical studies shall submit, for each clinical investigator who participated in a covered clinical study, either a certification described in paragraph (a)(1) of this section or a disclosure statement described in paragraph (a)(3) of this section.*
   1. *Certification: The applicant covered by this section shall submit for all clinical investigators (as defined in 54.2(d)), to whom the certification applies, a completed Form FDA 3454 attesting to the absence of financial interests and arrangements described in paragraph (a)(3) of this section. The form shall be dated and signed by the chief financial officer or other responsible corporate official or representative.*
   2. *If the certification covers less than all covered clinical data in the application, the applicant shall include in the certification a list of the studies covered by this certification.*
   3. *Disclosure Statement: For any clinical investigator defined in 54.2(d) for whom the applicant does not submit the certification described in paragraph (a)(1) of this section, the applicant shall submit a completed Form FDA 3455 disclosing completely and accurately the following:*
      i. *Any financial arrangement entered into between the sponsor of the covered study and the clinical investigator involved in the conduct of a covered clinical trial, whereby the value of the compensation to the clinical investigator for conducting the study could be influenced by the outcome of the study;*
      ii. *Any significant payments of other sorts from the sponsor of the covered study, such as a grant to fund ongoing research, compensation in the form of equipment, retainer for ongoing consultation, or honoraria;*
      iii. *Any proprietary interest in the tested product held by any clinical investigator involved in a study;*

iv. *Any significant equity interest in the sponsor of the covered study held by any clinical investigator involved in any clinical study; and*
v. *Any steps taken to minimize the potential for bias resulting from any of the disclosed arrangements, interests, or payments.*

b. *The clinical investigator shall provide to the sponsor of the covered study sufficient accurate financial information to allow the sponsor to submit complete and accurate certification or disclosure statements as required in paragraph (a) of this section. The investigator shall promptly update this information if any relevant changes occur in the course of the investigation or for 1 year following completion of the study.*
c. *Refusal to file application. FDA may refuse to file any marketing application described in paragraph (a) of this section that does not contain the information required by this section or a certification by the applicant that the applicant has acted with due diligence to obtain the information but was unable to do so and stating the reason.*

Section 505 of the Food Drug and Cosmetics Act ("the Act") describes three types of new drug applications: (i) an application that contains full reports of investigations of safety and effectiveness (section 505(b)(1)); (ii) an application that contains full reports of investigations of safety and effectiveness but where at least some of the information required for approval comes from studies not conducted by or for the applicant and for which the applicant has not obtained a right of reference (section 505(b)(2)); and (iii) an application that contains information to show that the proposed product is identical in active ingredient, dosage form, strength, route of administration, labeling, quality, performance characteristics, and intended use, among other things, to a previously approved product (section 505(j)). Note that a supplement to an application is a new drug application.

Section 506 of the Act allows the FDA grant accelerated approval for regenerative therapeutic products and directs the FDA to consider the unique characteristics of such therapies and provide a rationale for a determination of whether or not to grant accelerated approval.

Section 510(k) of the Act refers to the requirement for medical device manufacturers who must register with the FDA to notify the agency 90 days in advance of their intent to market a "substantially equivalent" device, also known as premarket notification.

Section 513 of the Act addresses medical device reclassification procedures.

Section 515 of the Act addresses the FDA's approval of medical device premarket approval applications.

Sponsors are required to submit a list of all clinical investigators conducting covered studies in their IND or IDE application (21 CFR Part 312.23(6)(iii)(b) and 21 CFR Part 812.20(b)(5), respectively).[3,4]

For each clinical investigator, the sponsor must provide certification or disclosure documentation as appropriate, unless that is not possible as indicated in 21 CFR Part 54.4: *Where the applicant acts with due diligence to obtain the information required in this section but is unable to do so, the applicant shall certify that despite the applicant's due diligence in attempting to obtain the information, the applicant was unable to obtain the information and shall include the reason.*[1]

The regulation defines and gives examples of disclosable interests including compensation based on study outcomes, equity and proprietary interests, and significant payments of other sorts (SPOOS) to the clinical investigator or institution. It is important to review these definitions carefully when completing the required certification or disclosure forms.

If sponsors intend to use a questionnaire to collect financial information from investigators, FDA recommends that they develop forms suited to that purpose. FORM FDA 3455 (Disclosure: Financial Interests and Arrangements of Clinical Investigators) *was designed for applicants to use to report financial information they collected from clinical investigators to FDA. It does not include the background information needed for clinical investigators to be aware of the financial information to be provided. For example, there is no statement that the reporting requirements apply to the spouse and dependent children as well as to the investigator; no information as to the dollar amounts triggering reporting of equity interests or SPOOS; and no statement that the investigator must report the details of the financial interests and arrangements, not just a statement, for example, of equity interest greater than $50,000. In addition, when there is more than one sponsor for financial disclosure purposes, the investigator should be apprised that the dollar amounts triggering reporting apply separately to each sponsor. This type of explanatory information should be provided to the clinical investigators to ensure that the financial disclosure information collected is as accurate and complete as possible.*[2]

An appendix in the guidance is provided for considerations for collecting financial disclosure information from clinical investigators.

All clinical investigators with no disclosable interests are listed together on Form FDA 3454 Certification: Financial Interests and Arrangements of Clinical Investigators and submitted to the agency.

For *each* clinical investigator with disclosable interests, Form FDA 3455 Disclosure: Financial Interests and Arrangements of Clinical Investigators is completed and submitted to the agency.

Compliance with 21 CFR Part 54.4(b) requires the clinical investigator to *promptly update the information if any relevant changes occur in the course of the investigation or for 1 year following completion of the study.*[1]

However, because the sponsor is obligated to collect the information, operationally, drug and biologic product sponsors typically remind clinical investigators of the updating requirements, or may request updated financial disclosure documentation on an annual basis. Many sponsors also review Form FDA 1572 from each participating clinical investigator to identify the clinical investigator and any listed subinvestigators from whom certification or disclosure of interests should be collected.

Because Form FDA 1572 is specific to drug regulatory compliance, it is not required for medical device studies. Device product sponsors generally use either an Investigator Agreement (IA) form or a protocol signature page to identify the clinical investigator for a given study site. The 1572 is an official FDA form, while IAs or protocol signature pages are typically sponsor-generated forms which incorporate similar information and requirements as the 1572. The other main difference between a 1572 and the IA, is that the IA references a commitment to device rather than drug regulatory compliance.

While the 1572 used for drug studies includes sections for identifying the clinical investigator and for listing additional subinvestigators, device sponsor-generated IAs and protocol signature pages are often only collected from the clinical investigator and may not include a list of subinvestigators.

Even with the use of a 1572, sponsors should review the clinical investigator delegation documentation at each research site to determine if the clinical investigator has assigned any subinvestigators from whom disclosure or certification information should be collected. The FDA may also review delegation documentation during an inspection.

Monitors should be trained to ensure that changes to the clinical investigator delegation of duties that identify either new or departing clinical investigators and/or subinvestigators are communicated for appropriate follow-up in obtaining current and future certification or disclosure documents, as well as updating the 1572 for drug studies.

AGENCY EVALUATION OF FINANCIAL INTERESTS

a. ***Evaluation of disclosure statement.*** *FDA will evaluate the information disclosed under 54.4(a)(2) about each covered clinical study in an application to determine the impact of any disclosed financial interests on the reliability of the study. FDA may consider both the size and nature of a disclosed financial interest (including the potential increase in the value of the interest if the product is approved) and steps that have been taken to minimize the potential for bias.*
b. ***Effect of study design.*** *In assessing the potential of an investigator's financial interests to bias a study, FDA will take into account the design and purpose of the study. Study designs that utilize such approaches as multiple investigators (most of whom do not have a disclosable interest), blinding, objective endpoints, or measurement of endpoints by someone other than the investigator may adequately protect against any bias created by a disclosable financial interest.*
c. ***Agency actions to ensure reliability of data.*** *If FDA determines that the financial interests of any clinical investigator raise a serious question about the integrity of the data, FDA will take any action it deems necessary to ensure the reliability of the data including:*
   1. *Initiating agency audits of the data derived from the clinical investigator in question;*
   2. *Requesting that the applicant submit further analyses of data, e.g., to evaluate the effect of the clinical investigator's data on overall study outcome;*
   3. *Requesting that the applicant conduct additional independent studies to confirm the results of the questioned study; and*
   4. *Refusing to treat the covered clinical study as providing data that can be the basis for an agency action.*

21 CFR Part 54 does not categorically prohibit clinical investigators with disclosable financial interests or arrangements from participating in covered clinical trial, but it does require applicants to submit a list of clinical investigators who are full-time and part-time employees of the sponsor and to disclose or certify certain financial interests with respect to other clinical investigators so that the FDA can assess the possibility of bias. The type of financial interest or arrangement disclosed is important because some financial interests and arrangements are of greater concern than others when assessing the reliability of the data.

Should a sponsor choose to engage a clinical investigator that has a disclosable financial interest, the sponsor bears the burden of assuring the FDA that they have evaluated the potential for bias to be introduced and have taken effective steps to ensure that the potential for bias is eliminated. To follow is an example of such a situation, in which there was a disclosable financial interest of the clinical investigator that was successfully negotiated with the FDA.

A medical device sponsor conducted a pivotal study on a new indication for their commercially available durable medical device. One of their paid consultants, also a shareholder, was identified as the primary clinical investigator in a US-based multi-site study. The disclosable financial interests reported showed that the clinical investigator would profit from device sales as well as an increase in the value of company stocks owned if the study was successful and additional indications were added to the device's already legally marketed use. Being intimately familiar with the device technology and a subject matter expert in the field of study, this clinical investigator was been assigned to adjudicate, i.e., perform an independent review and assessment of unanticipated adverse device effects (UADEs) for all clinical investigators participating in the study. Under US medical device regulations, UADEs are only reportable if they are both unanticipated and assessed to be related to the investigational device. The FDA objected to this approach due to the significant risk of introducing bias in this situation. If the clinical investigator assessed the events as not potentially related to the investigational use of the device, the event would not be reportable. Under these circumstances, the FDA indicated the data from the study could be rejected.

The sponsor addressed the potential for bias by not only assigning a different clinical investigator with no disclosable financial relationship to re-adjudicate all UADEs, but also to re-review and adjudicate all adverse experiences that occurred at the center of the clinical investigator with the financial interest. The FDA was satisfied with the solution and accepted the data from the clinical investigator with financial interest under these circumstances.

RECORDKEEPING AND RECORD RETENTION

a. ***Financial records of clinical investigators to be retained.*** *An applicant who has submitted a marketing application containing covered clinical studies shall keep on file certain information pertaining to the financial interests of clinical investigators who conducted studies on which the application relies and who are not full-time or part-time employees of the applicant, as follows:*

1. *Complete records showing any financial interest or arrangement as described in 54.4(a)(3)(i) paid to such clinical investigators by the sponsor of the covered study.*
2. *Complete records showing significant payments of other sorts, as described in 54.4(a)(3)(ii), made by the sponsor of the covered clinical study to the clinical investigator.*
3. *Complete records showing any financial interests held by clinical investigators as set forth in 54.4(a)(3)(iii) and (a)(3)(iv).*

b. ***Requirements for maintenance of clinical investigators' financial records.***

1. *For any application submitted for a covered product, an applicant shall retain records as described in paragraph (a) of this section for 2 years after the date of approval of the application.*
2. *The person maintaining these records shall, upon request from any properly authorized officer or employee of FDA, at reasonable times, permit such officer or employee to have access to and copy and verify these records.*

Sponsors may need to retain records of clinical investigators' financial records for much longer than 2 years, as the retention period extends 2 years beyond the approval of an application. And because the sponsor may not be the applicant, there may be uncertainty about the date of approval or retention period.

The Trial Master File for a given trial may house financial information relevant to the conduct of the trial, but typically disclosable financial interests, such as Form FDA 3455 are not included. Therefore, sponsors should have written procedures for controlling and archiving these documents to ensure their availability at the time future applications may be made to the FDA.

REFERENCES

1. Federal Register (2013, February 1). *21 CFR Part 54 Financial Disclosure by Clinical Investigators: Guidance for Clinical Investigators, Industry, and FDA Staff.* Code of Federal Regulations. Retrieved October 4, 2023, from https://www.federalregister.gov/documents/1998/02/02/98-2407/financial-disclosure-by-clinical-investigators
2. FDA (2013, February 1). *Financial Disclosure by Clinical Investigators: Guidance for Clinical Investigators, Industry, and FDA Staff.* FDA.gov. Retrieved October 4, 2023, from https://www.fda.gov/regulatory-information/search-fda-guidance-documents/financial-disclosure-clinical-investigators
3. Federal Register (1987, March 19). *21 CFR Part 312 Investigational New Drug Application.* Code of Federal Regulations. Retrieved October 4, 2023, from https://www.federalregister.gov/documents/1998/02/02/98-2407/financial-disclosure-by-clinical-investigators
4. Federal Register (1980, January 18). *21 CFR Part 812 Investigational Device Exemptions.* Code of Federal Regulations. Retrieved October 4, 2023, from https://www.federalregister.gov/documents/1998/02/02/98-2407/financial-disclosure-by-clinical-investigators

8 Institutional Review Boards

Aurea Flores

Author's Note

For the purposes of this chapter, the terms research, clinical investigation, clinical research investigation, and clinical trial are interchangeable.

ABBREVIATIONS

DHHS	Department of Health & Human Services
DMC	Data Monitoring Committee
DSMB	Data Safety Monitoring Board
DSMC	Data Safety Monitoring Committee
FDA	Food and Drug Administration
FWA	Federalwise Assurance
HDE	Humanitarian Device Exemption
IEC	Institutional Ethics Committee
IND	Investigational New Drug
IDE	Investigational Device Exemption
IRB	Institutional Review Board
NIH	National Institutes of Health
OHRP	Office of Human Research Protection
PHS	Public Health Services

HISTORY

Introduction

The history of clinical trials is not one to be most proud of. As clinical trial professionals, we can learn from past mistakes, with an emphasis on doing right for all humankind now and in the future, by conducting ethical clinical trials.

Ethics is defined as the moral principles that govern a person's behavior or the conduct of an activity. Institutional Review Boards main focus is to oversee the ethical conduct of clinical trials. In countries outside the United States of America, IRBs are also referred to as Institutional Ethics Committees (IECs). For the purpose of clinical research investigations and clinical trials, IRBs and IECs are interchangeable.

 DOI: 10.1201/9781003407010-8

Nuremberg Code

During the late 1930s to mid-1940s, Nazi-led government scientists conducted experiments in their prisons, health facilities, and concentration camps using children and adults. Most of these experiments utilized members of society that the Nazis considered expendable and/or subhuman. As a result, these individuals had no rights and were not involved in decisions about whether they wanted to participate or not in these experiments. In some cases, the experiments involved unethical procedures that caused pain and discomfort and, in some cases, led to death. The risks of these experiments to the participants were never taken into account, only the potential benefits as to how the results would help with Nazi ideology and war efforts.

After World War II ended, the United States indicted 23 defendants in connection with the experimentation in concentration camps during World War II. It is believed that that was only the tip of the iceberg. Many more would have to be involved for such a conspiracy against humanity to have lasted as long as it did. Nonetheless, the trial took place from December 1946 to August 1947. Different from the original Nuremberg trial, this trial was conducted by the US military courts instead of the Internal Military Tribunal, yet the trial was conducted in the same court, the Palace of Justice in Nuremberg.

The court's verdict from the judges contained ten points and was later referred to as the Nuremberg Code. These points stressed the importance of obtaining consent from prospective participants free of force, deceit, duress, or other ulterior forms of coercion. Additionally, it integrated the Hippocratic oath of no harm into clinical research. The ten points are summarized below:

- The voluntary consent of the human subject is absolutely essential.
- The experiment should be designed to yield fruitful results for the good of society that cannot be procured by other means.
- The experiment should be designed and based on the results of experimen tation in animals and knowledge of the natural history of the disease or condition, whose anticipated results justify the conduct of the trial.
- The experiment should be conducted in such a manner as to avoid all unnecessary physical and mental suffering and injury.
- No experiment should be conducted where there is a reason to believe that death or disabling injury will occur.
- The risk resulting from participation in the experimentation should never exceed the risk encountered by the population afflicted with the disease/condition being studied in the normal procurement of medical treatment.
- The experiment should ensure that there are proper facilities to protect the trial participant against even the most remote possibilities of injury, disability, or death.
- The experiment should only be conducted by scientifically qualified people. The highest degree of skill and care should be required through all stages of the trial by those who conduct or engage in it.

- The trial participant should be at liberty to bring their participation in the trial to an end if he/she has reached the decision that continuation of his/her participation in the trials seems impossible.
- The scientist in charge of the trial must be prepared to terminate the trial at any stage if he/she has probable cause to believe, in his/her judgment, that the continuation of the trial is likely to result in injury, disability, or death of the trial participant.

Unfortunately, little change came as a result of the Nuremberg Code.

Declaration of Helsinki

In 1964, the World Medical Association wrote the Declaration of Helsinki, integrating the ten points from the Nuremberg Code. Over the years, this document has been updated several times, with the last version in October 2013 at the time of this publication. The Declaration of Helsinki was developed as a statement of ethical principles for medical research involving humans all around the world. Together, the Declaration of Helsinki and the Belmont Report establish the roadmap for conducting and overseeing clinical trials.

Belmont Report

From 1932 to 1972, the United States Public Health Services sponsored the Tuskegee Study of Untreated Syphilis in the Negro Male, also referred to as the Tuskegee Syphilis Study. The original research question that the study was trying to answer was not necessarily incorrect. At the time (early 1930s), the medical profession still believed that Black individuals were different from Caucasian individuals at all levels regarding not only status but also anatomy and pathophysiology. Healthcare was provided separately among the races, with the belief that the races must not be combined. Even interracial blood transfusions were not allowed for fear of reactions to the recipient and the mixing of the races. Therefore, understanding the disease of syphilis, among others, in the Black population would have shown, as we now know, that the disease course is similar to that of Caucasians and would have led to a better understanding of other races'/ethnicities health. The ethical issues with this study were several. Even though at the start of the trial participants were receiving the treatment at the time (mercury-based), there were risks to procedures that were not properly discussed, such as lumbar punctures (spinal taps), and proper informed consent was not obtained. In fact, participants were given the impression that they could not refuse participation. Additionally, the trial used inducement in the form of payment for participation, taking advantage of the participants' financial situation. Finally, once penicillin became available and was found to be highly effective in treating syphilis, the study was continued as it was originally designed, instead of st opping the study and offering the treatment to those participants who were able to receive it. The study continued with the objective of seeing the course of the disease to its inevitable endpoint: death.

Nowadays, such decisions are considered unethical, and it is the responsibility of the IRB to suspend the trial and ensure that participants' safety, welfare, and rights are protected any time new scientific information becomes available, such as effective treatments or unacceptable toxicity that would place participants at unnecessary risks of harm.

The Tuskegee Syphilis Study continued for over 40 years under different directors and personnel. In 1972, there was a leak to the press, which brought it to the attention of the public at large and the Public Health Services (PHS) Agency. The study was then terminated, and Congressional hearings were conducted to investigate.

As a result of the investigation, Congress passed the National Research Act, and a commission (National Commission for the Protection of Human Subjects in Biomedical and Behavioral Research) was created to study and create regulations governing study conduct in humans. Additionally, the United States Department of Health and Human Services created the Office of Human Research Protections (OHRP) to oversee participant protection in clinical trials.

The Commission created a report: *Belmont Report: Ethical Principles and Guidelines for the Protection of Human Subjects of Research, Report of the National Commission for the Protection of Human Subjects of Biomedical and Behavioral Research,* commonly referred to as the Belmont Report.

The Belmont Report establishes three fundamental ethical principles for using humans for research. These are:

- **Respect for Persons** – It is important to protect the autonomy of individuals, to treat them with respect, and to allow them to provide consent free of force and coercion (similar to point #1 of the Nuremberg Code).
- **Beneficence** – Do not harm by maximizing the benefits while minimizing the risks to the participants.
- **Justice** – Equal distribution of benefits to potential participants without targeting a particular group because they are considered expendable or subhuman.

The Belmont Report is referenced by all Institutional Review Boards in their reviews of clinical trials (see below).

Together, the Declaration of Helsinki and the Belmont Report establish the roadmap for conducting and overseeing clinical trials and the framework for Institutional Review Boards.

Havasupai Tribe Diabetes Project and Genetic Research

Between 1990 and 1994, the Diabetes Project led by researchers at Arizona State University, collected DNA samples from approximately 400 Havasupai tribe members. The stated intent of the research was to understand why more than half of Havasupai adults suffered from type 2 diabetes mellitus. The Diabetes Project included education about diabetes, the collection and testing of blood samples, and genetic testing to assess the association between genetics and diabetes disease. Prospective participants were approached and explained the trial verbally. If agreed, they were then presented with a written informed consent document. Although the consent document stated that the samples would be used for research on "behavioral/

medical problems," tribe members were told that their samples would be used specifically for genetic studies on diabetes. Initial studies failed to find a genetic link with type 2 diabetes mellitus. The samples were stored, subsequently used in other ongoing genetic studies, and distributed to researchers for other unrelated studies. These subsequent studies were conducted after receiving IRB approval and included studies on diabetes and schizophrenia. Mental illness is highly stigmatized in the Havasupai culture, and tribe members were made aware of the use of their specimens; they asserted that they would not have consented to such research had they been properly informed.

As a result, clinical investigations involving Native American individuals must first obtain the formal, written approval of the appropriate tribal government(s). Additionally, there are specific tribal IRBs to oversee research for specific Native American tribes. It is important for any investigator planning clinical research involving Native American individuals to understand and comply with the appropriate regulatory requirements for conducting clinical investigations involving members of Native American tribes.

Subpart A – General Provisions

21 CFR Part 56.101 Scope.

a. *This part contains the general standards for the composition, operation, and responsibility of an Institutional Review Board (IRB) that reviews clinical investigations regulated by the Food and Drug Administration under sections 505(i) and 520(g) of the act, as well as clinical investigations that support applications for research or marketing permits for products regulated by the Food and Drug Administration, including foods, including dietary supplements, that bear a nutrient content claim or a health claim, infant formulas, food and color additives, drugs for human use, medical devices for human use, biological products for human use, and electronic products. Compliance with this part is intended to protect the rights and welfare of human subjects involved in such investigations.*
b. *References in this part to regulatory sections of the Code of Federal Regulations are to chapter I of title 21, unless otherwise noted.*

[46 FR 8975, Jan. 27, 1981, as amended at 64 FR 399, Jan. 5, 1999; 66 FR 20599, Apr. 24, 2001]

21 CFR Part 56.102 Definitions.

As used in this part:

a. *Act means the Federal Food, Drug, and Cosmetic Act, as amended (secs. 201–902, 52 Stat. 1040 et seq., as amended (21 U.S.C. 321–392)).*
b. *Application for research or marketing permit includes:*
   1. *A color additive petition, described in part 71.*
   2. *Data and information regarding a substance submitted as part of the procedures for establishing that a substance is generally recognized as safe for a use which results or may reasonably be expected to result,*

directly or indirectly, in its becoming a component or otherwise affecting the characteristics of any food, described in § 170.35.

3. *A food additive petition, described in part 171.*
4. *Data and information regarding a food additive submitted as part of the procedures regarding food additives permitted to be used on an interim basis pending additional study, described in § 180.1.*
5. *Data and information regarding a substance submitted as part of the procedures for establishing a tolerance for unavoidable contaminants in food and food-packaging materials, described in section 406 of the act.*
6. *An investigational new drug application, described in part 312 of this chapter.*
7. *A new drug application, described in part 314.*
8. *Data and information regarding the bioavailability or bioequivalence of drugs for human use submitted as part of the procedures for issuing, amending, or repealing a bioequivalence requirement, described in part 320.*
9. *Data and information regarding an over-the-counter drug for human use submitted as part of the procedures for classifying such drugs as generally recognized as safe and effective and not misbranded, described in part 330.*
10. *An application for a biologics license, described in part 601 of this chapter.*
11. *Data and information regarding a biological product submitted as part of the procedures for determining that licensed biological products are safe and effective and not misbranded, as described in part 601 of this chapter.*
12. *An Application for an Investigational Device Exemption, described in part 812.*
13. *Data and information regarding a medical device for human use submitted as part of the procedures for classifying such devices, described in part 860.*
14. *Data and information regarding a medical device for human use submitted as part of the procedures for establishing, amending, or repealing a standard for such device, described in part 861.*
15. *An application for premarket approval of a medical device for human use, described in section 515 of the act.*
16. *A product development protocol for a medical device for human use, described in section 515 of the act.*
17. *Data and information regarding an electronic product submitted as part of the procedures for establishing, amending, or repealing a standard for such products, described in section 358 of the Public Health Service Act.*
18. *Data and information regarding an electronic product submitted as part of the procedures for obtaining a variance from any electronic product performance standard, as described in § 1010.4.*

19. *Data and information regarding an electronic product submitted as part of the procedures for granting, amending, or extending an exemption from a radiation safety performance standard, as described in § 1010.5.*
20. *Data and information regarding an electronic product submitted as part of the procedures for obtaining an exemption from notification of a radiation safety defect or failure of compliance with a radiation safety performance standard, described in subpart D of part 1003.*
21. *Data and information about a clinical study of an infant formula when submitted as part of an infant formula notification under section 412(c) of the Federal Food, Drug, and Cosmetic Act.*
22. *Data and information submitted in a petition for a nutrient content claim, described in § 101.69 of this chapter, and for a health claim, described in § 101.70 of this chapter.*
23. *Data and information from investigations involving children submitted in a new dietary ingredient notification, described in § 190.6 of this chapter.*

c. *Clinical investigation means any experiment that involves a test article and one or more human subjects, and that either must meet the requirements for prior submission to the Food and Drug Administration under section 505(i) or 520(g) of the act, or need not meet the requirements for prior submission to the Food and Drug Administration under these sections of the act, but the results of which are intended to be later submitted to, or held for inspection by, the Food and Drug Administration as part of an application for a research or marketing permit. The term does not include experiments that must meet the provisions of part 58, regarding nonclinical laboratory studies. The terms research, clinical research, clinical study, study, and clinical investigation are deemed to be synonymous for purposes of this part.*
d. *Emergency use means the use of a test article on a human subject in a life-threatening situation in which no standard acceptable treatment is available, and in which there is not sufficient time to obtain IRB approval.*
e. *Human subject means an individual who is or becomes a participant in research, either as a recipient of the test article or as a control. A subject may be either a healthy individual or a patient.*
f. *Institution means any public or private entity or agency (including Federal, State, and other agencies). The term facility as used in section 520(g) of the act is deemed to be synonymous with the term institution for purposes of this part.*
g. *Institutional Review Board (IRB) means any board, committee, or other group formally designated by an institution to review, to approve the initiation of, and to conduct periodic review of, biomedical research involving human subjects. The primary purpose of such review is to assure the protection of the rights and welfare of the human subjects. The term has the same meaning as the phrase institutional review committee as used in section 520(g) of the act.*
h. *Investigator means an individual who actually conducts a clinical investigation (i.e., under whose immediate direction the test article is administered or*

dispensed to, or used involving, a subject) or, in the event of an investigation conducted by a team of individuals, is the responsible leader of that team.

i. *Minimal risk means that the probability and magnitude of harm or discomfort anticipated in the research are not greater in and of themselves than those ordinarily encountered in daily life or during the performance of routine physical or psychological examinations or tests.*
j. *Sponsor means a person or other entity that initiates a clinical investigation, but that does not actually conduct the investigation, i.e., the test article is administered or dispensed to, or used involving, a subject under the immediate direction of another individual. A person other than an individual (e.g., a corporation or agency) that uses one or more of its own employees to conduct an investigation that it has initiated is considered to be a sponsor (not a sponsor-investigator), and the employees are considered to be investigators.*
k. *Sponsor-investigator means an individual who both initiates and actually conducts, alone or with others, a clinical investigation, i.e., under whose immediate direction the test article is administered or dispensed to, or used involving, a subject. The term does not include any person other than an individual, e.g., it does not include a corporation or agency. The obligations of a sponsor-investigator under this part include both those of a sponsor and those of an investigator.*
l. *Test article means any drug for human use, biological product for human use, medical device for human use, human food additive, color additive, electronic product, or any other article subject to regulation under the act or under sections 351 or 354–360F of the Public Health Service Act.*
m. *IRB approval means the determination of the IRB that the clinical investigation has been reviewed and may be conducted at an institution within the constraints set forth by the IRB and by other institutional and Federal requirements.*

[46 FR 8975, Jan. 27, 1981, as amended at 54 FR 9038, Mar. 3, 1989; 56 FR 28028, June 18, 1991; 64 FR 399, Jan. 5, 1999; 64 FR 56448preview citation details, Oct. 20, 1999; 65 FR 52302, Aug. 29, 2000; 66 FR 20599, Apr. 24, 2001; 74 FR 2368, Jan. 15, 2009]

The scope and definitions as defined in the CFR are provided for completeness since no interpretation of them is required,

IRB COMPOSITION

21 CFR Part 56.107 IRB Membership

a. *Each IRB shall have at least five members with varying backgrounds to promote complete and adequate review of research activities commonly conducted by the institution. The IRB shall be sufficiently qualified through the experience and expertise of its members and the diversity of the members, including consideration of race, gender, cultural backgrounds, and* *sensitivity to such issues as community attitudes, to promote respect for its advice and counsel in safeguarding the rights and welfare of human subjects. In addition to possessing the professional competence necessary to review the specific research activities, the IRB shall be able to ascertain the acceptability of proposed research in terms of institutional commitments and regulations, applicable law, and standards of professional conduct and practice. * * * The IRB shall therefore include persons knowledgeable in these areas. If an IRB regularly reviews research that involves a vulnerable category of subjects, such as children, prisoners, pregnant women, or handicapped or mentally disabled persons, consideration shall be given to the inclusion of one or more individuals who are knowledgeable about and experienced in working with those subjects.*

b. *Every nondiscriminatory effort will be made to ensure that no IRB consists entirely of men or entirely of women, including the institution's consideration of qualified persons of both sexes, so long as no selection is made to the IRB on the basis of gender. No IRB may consist entirely of members of one profession.*
c. *Each IRB shall include at least one member whose primary concerns are in the scientific area and at least one member whose primary concerns are in nonscientific areas.*
d. *Each IRB shall include at least one member who is not otherwise affiliated with the institution and who is not part of the immediate family of a person who is affiliated with the institution.*
e. *No IRB may have a member participate in the IRB's initial or continuing review of any project in which the member has a conflicting interest, except to provide information requested by the IRB.*
f. *An IRB may, in its discretion, invite individuals with competence in special areas to assist in the review of complex issues which require expertise beyond or in addition to that available on the IRB. These individuals may not vote with the IRB.*

All IRBs must have a chairperson. IRBs must be composed of at least five members, including the chair. The IRB must contain at least one member whose primary area of interest is NOT in the medical sciences, such as a community member.

For IRBs, which are part of organizations such as academic centers, health systems, etc., at least one member must be independent of the organization. This member could be a community member or an independent medical professional.

Other potential members are: a member of legal counsel, who may or may not vote, but is present at meetings and available to provide legal advice when required; and ad-hoc members who are included in discussions to provide expertise in specific topics but are not voting members.

Large organizations may have several IRBs dedicated to different types of clinical research. Each IRB has its own chair and membership and operates independently of each other. All IRBs within the organization then fall under an organizational umbrella usually referred to as the Human Research Protection Office or equivalent. Examples of dedicated IRBs include:

- Oncology IRB
- Psychosocial IRB
- Pediatric IRB
- Tribal IRB

Ancillary Committee Reviews

Some organizations, as well as some clinical trials, require review of the research by other committees in addition to those separate from the IRB. These committees, independently from the sponsor and IRB, may review the feasibility and scientific validity of the research, and/or the clinical trial data (safety and efficacy). Reports from these committees are forwarded to the IRB for consideration. Ultimately, it is the review and approval of the clinical investigation by the IRB that allows the study to open to enroll participants and to continue until its completion, with amendments as needed throughout the trial lifecycle.

Pre-IRB Review Committees

Scientific Review Committees – These committees are comprised of stakeholders within the investigator's organization who have scientific expertise in a specific area of science. Each organization must have a charter detailing the committee composition, frequency of meetings, responsibilities, timelines for submission, and record-keeping. This type of committee usually includes a biostatistician.

Feasibility – Organizations may convene committees to evaluate trial feasibility for specific resources or for safety evaluation. These committees may meet on an ad-hoc basis. An example is the Radiological Safety Committee/Equivalent, which may review the use of radio-isotopes in the organization. It is important for investigators to be aware of any required ancillary committee reviews prior to IRB to ensure there is no delay in IRB review.

Concomitant Review with IRB

Institutional Biosafety Committee (IBC) – These committees were originally established under the National Institutes of Health (NIH) Guidelines to provide local review and oversight of investigations involving recombinant or synthetic nucleic acid molecules, e.g., vectors, viruses, cells, etc., to ensure proper biosafety practices and containment principles for handling these molecules. Review and approval by a fully convened IBC are required before a clinical investigation involving recombinant or synthetic nucleic acid molecules can be opened for enrollment. IBC is independent of IRB. Their initial reviews can take place in parallel, and often these committees communicate their decisions to each other.

Post-IRB Review Committees

Data Safety Monitoring Board/Committee (DSMB/DSMC/DMC) – These types of committees are independent from the organization, sponsor and any other trial-related stakeholder. DSMB/DSMC/DMC are convened by the trial sponsor and comprise individuals with pertinent expertise to review regularly accumulating data from one or more ongoing clinical trials. The committee members must not have conflicts of interest with the organization/sponsor/other whose trial they are overseeing. DSMB/DSMC/DMC are recommended, not mandated, for trials of any size that compare rates of mortality or major morbidity. The committee must have a charter detailing the committee's composition, frequency of meetings, and responsibilities. In addition, one of the members must be a biostatistician not involved with the design of the trial(s) under committee oversight. These committees usually have 2 parts to each session: an open session where the data and results are presented and discussed, and a closed session where the committee members discuss further and come to a decision: continue the trial as is, require amendments, close enrollment, or suspend/terminate the trial. The committee decision is provided in writing and submitted to the IRB of record for its consideration and files.

Endpoint Assessment/Adjudication Committee, Also Referred to as Clinical Events Committee (CEC) – This type of committee is also convened by the trial sponsor for certain trials to review important endpoints to determine whether the endpoints are meeting protocol-specific criteria. The members must have pertinent expertise and be independent from the sponsor/investigator organizations. This committee is particularly valuable when endpoints are subjective and/or require the application of complex definitions. The committee reviewers maintain an impartial and effective decision by usually being masked as to whether the trial arm is blinded or not. The committee must have a charter detailing its composition, frequency of meetings, and responsibilities. One member must be a biostatistician not involved with the design of the trial(s) under committee oversight. The recommendations are provided in writing and submitted to the IRB of record in a timely manner, per IRB policies and procedures and committee charters.

IRB Procedures

21 CFR Part 56.108 IRB Functions and Operations

In order to fulfill the requirements of these regulations, each IRB shall:

a. *Follow written procedures:*
   1. *for conducting its initial and continuing review of research and for reporting its findings and actions to the investigator and the institution;*
   2. *for determining which projects require review more often than annually and which projects need verification from sources other than the investigator that no material changes have occurred since previous IRB reviews;*

   3. *for ensuring prompt reporting to the IRB of changes in research activity; and*
   4. *for ensuring that changes in approved research, during the period for which IRB approval has already been given, may not be initiated without IRB review and approval except where necessary to eliminate apparent immediate hazards to human subjects.*

b. *Follow written procedures for ensuring prompt reporting to the IRB, appropriate institutional officials, and the Food and Drug Administration of:*
   1. *Any unanticipated problems involving risks to human subjects or others;*
   2. *any instance of serious or continuing noncompliance with these regulations or the requirements or determinations of the IRB; or*
   3. *any suspension or termination of IRB approval.*

c. *Except when an expedited review procedure is used (see § 56.110), review proposed research at convened meetings at which a majority of the members of the IRB are present, including at least one member whose primary concerns are in nonscientific areas. In order for the research to be approved, it shall receive the approval of a majority of those members present at the meeting.*

IRBs must have written policies and procedures to govern their operations to ensure compliance with all applicable laws and regulations. Sponsors and investigators must be familiar with their IRB record policies and procedures in order to better communicate.

All IRBs must provide a list of their members with their qualifications, including their curriculum vitae, contact information, affiliations, financial disclosures, and managing any conflicts of interest. Additionally, IRBs must possess and provide a Federalwide Assurance (FWA) number. A FWA is the documentation of a commitment to comply with Federal regulations and maintain policies and procedures for the protection of human participants. A FWA is awarded and overseen by the Office of Human Research Protections (OHRP).

Subpart B—Organization and Personnel

§ 56.106 Registration.

a. *Who must register? Each IRB in the United States that reviews clinical investigations regulated by FDA under sections 505(i) or 520(g) of the act and each IRB in the United States that reviews clinical investigations that are intended to support applications for research or marketing permits for FDA-regulated products must register at a site maintained by the Department of Health and Human Services (HHS). (A research permit under section 505(i) of the act is usually known as an investigational new drug application (IND), while a research permit under section 520(g) of the act is usually known as an investigational device exemption (IDE).) An individual authorized to act on the IRB's behalf must submit the registration information. All other IRBs may register voluntarily.*

b. *What information must an IRB register? Each IRB must provide the following information:*

1. *The name, mailing address, and street address (if different from the mailing address) of the institution operating the IRB and the name, mailing address, phone number, facsimile number, and electronic mail address of the senior officer of that institution who is responsible for overseeing activities performed by the IRB;*
2. *The IRB's name, mailing address, street address (if different from the mailing address), phone number, facsimile number, and electronic mail address; each IRB chairperson's name, phone number, and electronic mail address; and the name, mailing address, phone number, facsimile number, and electronic mail address of the contact person providing the registration information.*
3. *The approximate number of active protocols involving FDA-regulated products reviewed. For purposes of this rule, an "active protocol" is any protocol for which an IRB conducted an initial review or a continuing review at a convened meeting or under an expedited review procedure during the preceding 12 months; and*
4. *A description of the types of FDA-regulated products (such as biological products, color additives, food additives, human drugs, or medical devices) involved in the protocols that the IRB reviews.*

c. *When must an IRB register? Each IRB must submit an initial registration. The initial registration must occur before the IRB begins to review a clinical investigation described in paragraph (a) of this section. Each IRB must renew its registration every 3 years. IRB registration becomes effective after review and acceptance by HHS.*

d. *Where can an IRB register? Each IRB may register electronically through http://ohrp.cit.nih.gov/efile. If an IRB lacks the ability to register electronically, it must send its registration information, in writing, to the Office of Good Clinical Practice, Office of Special Medical Programs, Food and Drug Administration, 10903 New Hampshire Ave., Bldg. 32, Rm. 5129, Silver Spring, MD 20993.*

e. *How does an IRB revise its registration information? If an IRB's contact or chairperson information changes, the IRB must revise its registration information by submitting any changes in that information within 90 days of the change. An IRB's decision to review new types of FDA-regulated products (such as a decision to review studies pertaining to food additives whereas the IRB previously reviewed studies pertaining to drug products) or to discontinue reviewing clinical investigations regulated by FDA is a change that must be reported within 30 days of the change. An IRB's decision to disband is a change that must be reported within 30 days of permanent cessation of the IRB's review of research. All other information changes may be reported when the IRB renews its registration. The revised information must be sent to FDA either electronically or in writing, in accordance with paragraph (d) of this section.*

[74 FR 2368, Jan. 15, 2009, as amended at 78 FR 16401, Mar. 15, 2013]

IRB Registration

45 CFR Part 46 Subpart E – Registration of Institutional Review Boards https://www.ecfr.gov/current/title-45/subtitle-A/subchapter-A/part-46/subpart-E) The IRB must provide to OHRP the following information for registration:

- Name, mailing address, and street address, if different from the mailing address, of the institution or organization operating the IRB
- Name, mailing address, and street address, if different from the mailing address, of the senior officer or head official of the institution or organization operating the IRB
- Name, mailing address and phone number, facsimile number, and electronic mail address of the contact person providing registration information
- Name, if any, assigned to the IRB by the institution, mailing address and phone number, facsimile number, and electronic mail address
- Name, phone number, and electronic mail address of the IRB chairperson
- Approximate numbers of:
  - All active protocols
  - Active protocols conducted or supported by the Department of Health and Human Services
- The approximate number of full-time positions devoted to IRB administrative activities

IRBs must also provide the full board meeting schedule with timelines for submissions. Coordinators/administrators are employed to initially receive and review all submissions prior to assigning reviewers. These include:

- Initial clinical investigational trial submissions
- Amendment submissions – may include amendments to the investigational plan (trial protocol), clarification letters, informed consent, participant-facing materials, and intervention information (e.g., investigator drug brochures, device information, etc.)
- Reportable events – may include adverse events, serious adverse events, unanticipated device effects, trial protocol violations/deviations, planned deviations, and IND safety reports
- Continuing review submissions
- Trial completion submissions

The IRB coordinators/administrators review the submissions for completeness, and if the submission is deficient, they will communicate with the submitter to address the deficiencies. Only when the submission is complete will the coordinator/administrator decide whether the clinical investigation will require Full Board, Expedited, Limited, or is Exempt from IRB review. These decisions are confirmed with the IRB chairperson.

IRBs must have procedures that detail the different types of reviews, such as Full Board, Limited, Expedited, Emergency/Compassionate, and Exempt. Additionally, they must have procedures to appeal IRB decisions. It is important for investigators, sites, sponsors, and sponsor representatives to be familiar with the IRB's record policies and procedures.

Examples of IRB Policies and Procedures include:

- IRB Charter
    - IRB Responsibilities
    - IRB Membership
    - IRB Voting
    - IRB Record Keeping
- Research Activities Subject to IRB Jurisdiction
- Initial Review
- Expedited Review
- Limited Review
- Exempt Research
- Single IRB Review
- Cooperative Research IRB Review
- Emergency Use of Test Articles
- Compassionate Use of Test Articles
- Humanitarian Use Devices
- Unanticipated Problems
- Revisions and Amendments Submissions and Review
- Continuing Review
- Suspension or Termination of IRB Approval of Research
- External Reporting
- Informed Consent
    - Parental Permission
    - Assent
    - Legally Authorize Representative
    - Reconsenting
    - Broad Consent
    - Electronic Informed Consent
- Protocol Deviation/Violation Reporting
- Conflicts of Interest and Investigator Certifications/Representations
- Privacy Review
- Allegations of Research Non-Compliance, Concerns, or Complaints

RESEARCH ACTIVITIES SUBJECT TO IRB REVIEW

Any activities that fall under the OHRP and/or FDA definitions of research are subject to IRB jurisdiction.

OHRP Definition of Research – a systematic investigation, including research development, testing, and evaluation, designed to develop or contribute to generalizable knowledge.

FDA Definition of Research – any experiment that involves a test article and one or more human subjects and that either must meet the requirements for prior submission to the FDA...or the results of which are intended to be later submitted to, or held for inspection by, the FDA as part of an application for a research or marketing permit. These include clinical investigations that required IND, IDE, and HDE, in addition to IND-exempt and IDE-exempt.

Any clinical investigation involving living individuals about whom an investigator conducting the research obtains: (i) data through intervention or interaction with the individual, or (ii) identifiable private information.

IRB review is required for any clinical investigation that falls under the definitions above, including prospective interventional (trials drugs/biologics/devices), prospective observational trials, and retrospective investigations evaluating private identifiable information.

IRB REVIEW TYPES

21 CFR Part 56.111 Criteria for IRB Approval of Research

a. *In order to approve research covered by these regulations, the IRB shall determine that all of the following requirements are satisfied:*
   1. *Risks to subjects are minimized:*
      i. *By using procedures which are consistent with sound research design and which do not unnecessarily expose subjects to risk, and*
      ii. *whenever appropriate, by using procedures already being performed on the subjects for diagnostic or treatment purposes.*
   2. *Risks to subjects are reasonable in relation to anticipated benefits, if any, to subjects and the importance of the knowledge that may be expected to result. In evaluating risks and benefits, the IRB should consider only those risks and benefits that may result from the research (as distinguished from risks and benefits of therapies that subjects would receive even if not participating in the research). The IRB should not consider possible long-range effects of applying knowledge gained in the research (for example, the possible effects of the research on public policy) as among those research risks that fall within the purview of its responsibility.*
   3. *Selection of subjects is equitable. In making this assessment, the IRB should take into account the purposes of the research and the setting in which the research will be conducted and should be particularly cognizant of the special problems of research involving vulnerable populations, such as children, prisoners, pregnant women, handicapped or mentally disabled persons, or economically or educationally disadvantaged persons.*
   4. *Informed consent will be sought from each prospective subject or the subject's legally authorized representative, in accordance with and to the extent required by part 50.*

5. *Informed consent will be appropriately documented, in accordance with and to the extent required by § 50.27.*
6. *Where appropriate, the research plan makes adequate provision for monitoring the data collected to ensure the safety of subjects.*
7. *Where appropriate, there are adequate provisions to protect the privacy of subjects and to maintain the confidentiality of data.*

b. *When some or all of the subjects, such as children, prisoners, pregnant women, handicapped or mentally disabled persons, or economically or educationally disadvantaged persons, are likely to be vulnerable to coercion or undue influence additional safeguards have been included in the study to protect the rights and welfare of these subjects.*

c. *In order to approve research in which some or all of the subjects are children, an IRB must determine that all research is in compliance with part 50, subpart D of this chapter.*

Full Board Review

A full board IRB review is required for all clinical trials involving exposing human participants to more than minimal risk.

Minimal risk is defined as the probability and magnitude of anticipated harm or discomfort, which are no greater in and on themselves than those ordinarily encountered in daily life or during the performance of routine physical or psychological examinations or tests.

Examples of instances where greater than minimal risk is involved include:

- Exposure to an investigational drug, biologic, or significant-risk medical device
- Clinical investigations including participant procedures outside of clinical care for the disease being evaluated.

For a favorable determination by the IRB, the clinical trial must find that:

- Informed consent sought from prospective participants is in compliance with applicable federal, state, and local regulations. Traditionally, IRBs have reviewed documents containing information about the trial to assist the prospective participant with making an informed decision as to whether to participate in the trial. However, nowadays, information for prospective participants may be provided in different media, such as video/audio recordings. The key is to comply with the intent of the Federal regulations regarding informed consent: inform and provide information about the trial in the most effective manner for the prospective participant to make an informed decision as to whether or not to participate in the research. Additionally, the age of majority and definitions of a legally authorized representative vary by state. Therefore, the IRBs must take these local requirements into consideration when reviewing informed consent materials and the process to obtain consent. This responsibility is in support of the Belmont Report Principle: Respect.

- **Risks to Participants are Minimized** – This process involves determining whether the procedures to be performed on participants are consistent with sound medical care and research design and do not unnecessarily expose participants to risk. For example, a clinical trial designed to evaluate a new investigational, non-FDA-approved drug in patients diagnosed with acute myelogenous leukemia requires a bone marrow aspiration and biopsy at baseline (before investigational drug treatment), within 2 weeks of completing investigational treatment, and every 3 months thereafter. A bone marrow aspiration and biopsy is an invasive procedure, but in the context of this clinical trial, it is consistent with the provision of care in this patient population without participation in a clinical trial. On the other hand, as was the case in the Tuskegee Syphilis Study, a lumbar puncture was required for all participants at specified intervals, even though it is not consistent with medical practice for all patients diagnosed with syphilis. Performing a lumbar puncture in this patient population exposed the participants to greater than minimal risk, and it was not indicated. Furthermore, risks to participants must be reasonable in relation to anticipated benefits. This responsibility is in support of the Belmont Report Principle: Beneficence.
- **Selection of Participants is Equitable** – the clinical trial should not enroll participants only from a particular group of individuals. For instance, Nazis performed experiments on populations they considered inferior: Jews, Roma, feeble-minded, homosexuals, and others. There are exceptions when the clinical trial enrolls participants from a particular group of individuals where the disease/conditions is only present in that patient population. This responsibility is in support of the Belmont Report Principle: Justice.

Clinical investigations involving children have additional considerations for the IRB. These include clinical investigations:

- involve no greater than minimal risk to the participants;
- if greater than minimal risk is involved, the clinical investigation must present the prospect of direct benefit to the participants;
- if greater than minimal risk is involved with no prospect of direct benefit, then the risk must present a minor increase over minimal risk to the participants;
- if the clinical investigation does not fall under the three bullet points above and therefore is not approvable, then it must present an opportunity to understand, prevent, or alleviate a serious problem affecting the health/ welfare of children in general;

Clinical investigations involving pregnant women or fetuses have additional consideration for the IRB:

- Pre-clinical studies have been completed in pregnant animals and clinical studies in non-pregnant women have been conducted to provide data for assessing potential risks to pregnant women and fetuses.

- The risk to the fetus is caused solely by interventions or procedures that hold out the prospect of direct benefit for the woman or the fetus; or, if there is no such prospect of benefit, the risk to the fetus is not greater than minimal, and the purpose of the research is the development of important biomedical knowledge that cannot be obtained by any other means.
- The clinical investigation holds out the prospect of direct benefit to the pregnant woman, the prospect of a direct benefit both to the pregnant woman and the fetus, or no prospect of benefit for the woman nor the fetus when the risk to the fetus is not greater than minimal, and the purpose of the research is the development of important biomedical knowledge that cannot be obtained by any other means.
- No inducements, monetary or otherwise, will be offered to terminate a pregnancy.
- Individuals engaged in the clinical investigation will have no part in any decisions as to the timing, method, or procedures used to terminate a pregnancy.
- Individuals engaged in the clinical investigation will have no part in determining the viability of a neonate.

Clinical investigations involving neonates have additional considerations for the IRB:

- Where scientifically appropriate, preclinical and clinical studies have been conducted and provide data for assessing potential risks to neonates.
- Individuals engaged in the clinical investigation will have no part in determining the viability of a neonate.
- For neonates of uncertain viability, the IRB must determine that the clinical investigation has the least possible risk to hold out the prospect of enhancing the probability of survival of the neonate to the point of viability. The purpose of the clinical investigation is the development of important biomedical knowledge that cannot be obtained by other means, and there will be no added risk to the neonate resulting from participation.
- For non-viable neonates, the IRB must determine that the clinical investigation does not involve vital functions maintained artificially; there is no termination of heartbeat or respiration; there is no added risk to the neonate resulting from participation; and the purpose of the clinical investigation is the development of important biomedical knowledge that cannot be obtained by other means.

The IRB may review clinical investigations involving prisoners, taking into consideration the following:

- Any possible advantages of the prisoner through his or her participation in the clinical investigation, when compared to the general living conditions, medical care, quality of food, amenities, and opportunity for earnings in the prison, are not of such magnitude that his or her ability to weigh the risks of the research against the value of such advantages in the limited choice environment of the prison is impaired,

- The risks involved in the research are commensurate with risks those would be accepted by non-prisoner volunteers.
- The procedures for the selection of participants within the prison are fair to all prisoners and immune from arbitrary intervention by prison authorities.
- Parole boards may not take into account a prisoner's participation in the clinical investigation in making decisions regarding parole, and prisoners are clearly informed in advance of their participation.
- Clinical investigations are designed to study the possible causes, effects, and processes of incarceration and criminal behavior.
- A clinical investigation must present no more than minimal risk and no more than inconvenience to the participant.
- Clinical investigations that study conditions particularly affecting prisoners as a class. Examples include clinical investigations on vaccines, hepatitis, and social and psychological problems such as alcoholism, drug addiction, and sexual assaults. Consultation with the Secretary of DHHS is required.
- Clinical investigations on practices that have the intent and reasonable probability of improving the health or well-being of the participant.

Furthermore, the IRB must ensure that additional safeguards are in place when clinical investigations include handicapped or mentally disabled individuals, economically or educationally disadvantaged individuals, and/or any other persons who are likely to be vulnerable to coercion or undue influence.

Clinical investigations involving the prospective evaluation of drugs, biologics, and significant-risk medical devices are subject to full board review. At least two IRB members are assigned to conduct the review on behalf of the IRB.

It is important to understand that the IRB reviewers are not necessarily experts in the disease/condition to be evaluated. Therefore, relying on the IRB reviewers to understand technical information contained within documents such as clinical trial protocols and/or Investigator Brochures may cause a delay in the review. For that purpose, IRB submissions are meant to explain the clinical investigation in simple terms for any member, regardless of their qualifications and background, to fully understand and be able to evaluate the risks and benefits for participants. It is important that the IRB application be completed with all appropriate details to assist the reviewers in their determination. At its core, the IRB represents prospective participants.

In order for a full board meeting to convene, it must have a majority of the members of the IRB present, including one member whose primary concern is in nonscientific areas. After each review, IRB members shall make motions for actions on behalf of the committee. In order for motions to carry forward, they must receive the approval of a majority of the IRB members present at the meeting.

Required Documents for IRB review

Documents to be reviewed by the IRB include, but are not limited to:

- Clinical investigational plan
- Informed consent, written documents, and assent materials
  - Informed consent and assent materials may include video and audio recordings
- **Participant-Facing Materials** – diaries questionnaires, surveys, others
- Investigator Brochures or current scientific information, prescribing information, package inserts, device information/labeling
- Marketing and advertising information to prospective participants
- **Compensation for Participation and/or Injury** – usually included in the informed consent materials
- Investigator qualifications (curriculum vitae, professional license, board certifications, good clinical practice training), financial disclosures, and conflicts of interest management plans, if applicable
- Any other clinical trial information to be provided to participants
- Any other documents that IRB procedures consider pertinent to the review

Legally Authorized Representatives (LAR)

An investigator may request the use of LAR for obtaining informed consent and making decisions on behalf of a participant. In these cases, the IRB reviewers will evaluate the method to ensure appropriate LARs are used based on state and local laws. LAR definitions vary by state. The use of LARs must be reviewed and approved by the IRB of record. Investigators may not use LARs to obtain consent and make decisions related to clinical trial participation on behalf of the participants without prior approval by the IRB of record.

Assent

Similarly, IRB reviewers shall evaluate the need for assent (verbal or written) as well as the age at which assent is required (verbal or written) for underage prospective participants (children and adolescents). These determinations shall be based on IRB procedures, which in turn should be compliant with applicable regulations (federal, state, and local). The age of consent varies by jurisdiction, and the investigator and IRB must be familiar with applicable laws to ensure compliance.

Cooperative Research

21 CFR Part 56.114 Cooperative Research

In complying with these regulations, institutions involved in multi-institutional studies may use joint review, reliance upon the review of another qualified IRB, or similar arrangements aimed at avoidance of duplication of effort.

Cooperative research is defined as a clinical trial conducted by more than one institution receiving federal funding or sponsored by a federal agency or department. The Revised Common Rule introduced the concept of single IRBs, which allows for one IRB to review a clinical trial conducted in multiple separate institutions. Each location may have a different principal investigator and clinical trial team responsible for the conduct of the clinical investigation at that site. There should be, however, one coordinating site that is responsible for aggregating data and information from each site to submit to the single IRB of record for initial review, amendments, reportable events, continuing review, and a close-out report. It is noteworthy that each institution must provide their own informed consent document(s) to comply with all applicable federal, state, and local laws and regulations.

The use of a single IRB may not be applicable when Native American individuals are involved in the research since a tribal IRB is required to review clinical investigations involving these participants.

Institutions, organizations, and sites whose clinical investigations are not subject to the Revised Common Rule may enter into agreements with other institutions, organizations, or sites for joint review of the research using a single IRB. The agreement, referred to as a Reliance Agreement, allows participating sites to rely on the review of another IRB. Additionally, the agreement dictates the responsibilities of the participating sites and the coordinating site related to applications and submissions to the single IRB of record.

The purpose behind the single IRB is to avoid duplication of effort, and it is the result of the 21st century Cures Act provisions to alleviate administrative burdens.

Non-English-Speaking Participants

The investigator may request document translation from a certified translator once the IRB approves the informed consent form(s) and other participant-facing materials. The procedure for a certified translation is for the translator to translate the document(s) from English to the desired language, and then for a second translator to translate back from the desired language to English. The original English translation must be congruent with the second English translation. The investigator is responsible for submitting the translated documents along with the certificate of translation to the IRB. The IRB shall acknowledge receipt, at which time the investigator may begin consenting participants with the translated documents, as applicable.

Expedited Review

21 CFR Part 56.110 Expedited Review Procedures for Certain Kinds of Research Involving No More Than Minimal Risk, and for Minor Changes in Approved Research

a. *The Food and Drug Administration has established and published in the Federal Register a list of categories of research that may be reviewed by the IRB through an expedited review procedure. The list will be amended, as appropriate, through periodic republication in the Federal Register.*
b. *An IRB may use the expedited review procedure to review either or both of the following:*
    1. *Some or all of the research appearing on the list and found by the reviewer(s) to involve no more than minimal risk,*
    2. *Minor changes in previously approved research during the period (of 1 year or less) for which approval is authorized. Under an expedited review procedure, the review may be carried out by the IRB chairperson or by one or more experienced reviewers designated by the IRB chairperson from among the members of the IRB. In reviewing the research, the reviewers may exercise all of the authorities of the IRB,*

except that the reviewers may not disapprove the research. A research activity may be disapproved only after review in accordance with the nonexpedited review procedure set forth in § 56.108(c).

c. *Each IRB which uses an expedited review procedure shall adopt a method for keeping all members advised of research proposals which have been approved under the procedure.*
d. *The Food and Drug Administration may restrict, suspend, or terminate an institution's or IRB's use of the expedited review procedure when necessary to protect the rights or welfare of subjects.*

Certain types of clinical investigations may be reviewed without full board review when they involve no more than minimal risk to participants. Additionally, minor changes to previously approved research may fall under expedited review. Upon review of the IRB application by the IRB coordinator/administrator, the clinical investigation may fall under expedited review. Under expedited review, the review may be carried out by the IRB chairperson or by one or more experienced IRB reviewers designated by the IRB chairperson from among the members of the IRB. In this case, the designated reviewer may approve the clinical investigation and share the decision at the next full board meeting. However, the designated reviewer may not disapprove of the clinical investigation, in which case the application must be brought to the full board for discussion and disposition.

The Revised Common Rule introduced the concept of limited IRB review of expedited clinical investigations, where the clinical investigation is not required to be reviewed after initial review and approval. In fact, once the application is approved, it is no longer required to be reviewed on an ongoing basis. Under limited review, the IRB must determine that the identity of participants from information to be obtained by the investigator cannot be readily ascertained directly or indirectly through identifiers. However, some IRBs may require at least an annual update provided by the investigator for the IRB to be informed when the clinical investigation is completed and is no longer active.

Emergency/Compassionate Research

21 CFR Part 312.54 Emergency research under 50.24 of this chapter

a. *The sponsor shall monitor the progress of all investigations involving an exception from informed consent under § 50.24 of this chapter. When the sponsor receives from the IRB information concerning the public disclosures required by § 50.24(a)(7)(ii) and (a)(7)(iii) of this chapter, the sponsor promptly shall submit to the IND file and to Docket Number 95S-0158 in the Dockets Management Staff (HFA-305), Food and Drug Administration, 5630 Fishers Lane, rm. 1061, Rockville, MD 20852, copies of the information that was disclosed, identified by the IND number.*
b. *The sponsor also shall monitor such investigations to identify when an IRB determines that it cannot approve the research because it does not meet the criteria in the exception in § 50.24(a) of this chapter or because of other relevant ethical concerns. The sponsor promptly shall provide this*

> *information in writing to FDA, investigators who are asked to participate in this or a substantially equivalent clinical investigation, and other IRB's that are asked to review this or a substantially equivalent investigation.*

Under expanded access (for emergency and compassionate research), the FDA may allow the use of an investigational treatment (drug, biologic, and/or device) for the treatment of an individual patient by a licensed physician. Emergency and compassionate use of investigational products do not fall under the definition of research. However, the patient must provide consent to receive the investigational intervention. The IRB is responsible for reviewing the clinical investigational plan, Investigator Brochure and/or device information, and informed consent document for compliance with 21 CFR Part 50 (Protection of Human Subjects). The review of the activity falls under expedited review, with at least an annual continuing review to ensure the patient's safety, welfare, and rights are protected.

Exempt Research

There are no exempt IRB reviews under the FDA. However, the Revised Common Rule updated and expanded on the categories for exemption from IRB review. Institutional IRBs, especially academic IRBs, do oversee exempt research.

Clinical investigations involving human subjects that fall into any of the categories below are exempt from IRB review. However, only the IRB can determine whether the clinical investigation falls under an exemption, and therefore the investigator must submit an application to the IRB. Clinical investigations overseen by the FDA do not allow exempt reviews. These clinical investigations are under INDs, IDEs, or HDEs and are always considered greater than minimal risk. For clinical investigations that are considered IND-exempt and/or IDE-exempt, the review may be full board or expedited based on the risk levels of participants. The IRB shall make that determination at the time of review of the application.

Exempt Categories

Educational Settings

These are clinical investigations conducted in established or commonly accepted educational settings, which specifically involve normal education practices that are not likely to adversely impact students' opportunity to learn required educational content or the assessment of educators who provide instruction. Examples include collecting data on instructional activities, techniques, strategies, and the effectiveness of such activities, techniques and strategies, as long as they do not interfere with the educational activities within those educational settings.

Educational Testing

These are clinical investigations that only include interactions involving educational tests (cognitive, diagnostic, aptitude, and achievement), survey procedures, interview procedures, or observation of public behavior (including visual or auditory recordings) as long as:

- The data obtained is recorded in such a manner that it is anonymous, and the identity of the participants cannot be readily ascertained.
- Disclosure of the participant's responses outside of the investigation would not reasonably place them at risk of criminal or civil liability or be damaging to the participants' financial standing, employability, educational advancement, or reputation.
- In the event that information obtained is recorded in such a manner that the identity of the individual can be readily ascertained, directly or through identifiers, the IRB must conduct a limited review to ascertain the investigator's procedures to protect participants' privacy and confidentiality of the data. In this case, the investigator must show the procedures to maintain privacy and confidentiality in order for the investigation to be exempt. In some instances, the IRB may decide that the clinical investigation may fall under expedited review.

Benign Behavioral Interventions

Benign behavioral interactions are brief in duration, harmless, painless, not physically invasive, not likely to have a significant adverse lasting impact on the participants, and the investigator has no reason to think the participants will find the interventions offensive or embarrassing.

Clinical investigations involving benign behavioral interventions in conjunction with the collection of data from an adult through verbal or written responses (including data entry) or audiovisual recording are exempt as long as:

- The information is recorded by the investigator in such a manner that the identity of the participants cannot be readily ascertained, either directly or through identifiers.
- Disclosure of the participant's responses outside of the investigation would not reasonably place them at risk of criminal or civil liability or be damaging to the participants' financial standing, employability, educational advancement, or reputation.
- In the event that information obtained is recorded in such a manner that the identity of the individual can be readily ascertained directly or through identifiers, the IRB must conduct a limited review to ascertain the provisions to protect participants' privacy and confidentiality of the data. In this case, the investigator must show the procedures to maintain privacy and confidentiality in order for the investigation to be exempt. In some instances, the IRB may decide that the clinical investigation may fall under expedited review.

Additionally, if the investigation involves participant deception regarding the nature or purposes of the investigation, the clinical investigation is not exempt from IRB review and oversight, unless the participant authorizes the deception through a prospective agreement to participate where they will be unaware of or misled regarding the nature or purposes of the investigation.

Secondary Research for Which Consent Is Not Required

This applies to investigations where consent is not required and the investigation shall use identifiable private information or identifiable biospecimens. In order for this type of investigation to be exempt, it must meet one of the following criteria:

- Identifiable private information or identifiable biospecimens are publicly available;
- The data, including biospecimens, must be recorded in such a manner that the identity of the participant cannot be readily ascertained directly or through identifiers;
- The information collected and analyzed involves the use of identifiable health information when the use is regulated by 45 CFR Part 160 and 164, subparts A and E (HIPAA), for the purposes of healthcare operations, research, or public health activities. Please refer to the chapter: Protected Health Information and Privacy in Clinical Trials (HIPAA);
- The investigation is conducted by, or on behalf of a Federal department or agency using government-generated or government-collected information obtained for non-research activities.

Federally-Supported Research

This research includes investigations and projects that are conducted or supported by a Federal department or agency, or are otherwise subject to the approval of the agency/department heads. These investigations are designed to study, evaluate, improve, or examine public benefit or service programs, procedures for obtaining benefits or services under those programs, possible changes or alternatives to those programs or procedures, or methods of payment for benefits or services under those programs. Examples include, but are not limited to, internal studies by Federal employees, studies under contracts or consulting arrangements, cooperative agreements, or grants.

Taste and Food Quality Studies

Investigations to evaluate taste, food quality, and consumer acceptance are exempt if:

- The investigation involves wholesome foods without additives that are to be consumed by the participants, or
- The investigation involves food that contains a food ingredient at or below the level and for a use found to be safe by the Food and Drug Administration, or
- The investigation involves food with agricultural chemicals or environmental contaminants at or below the level found to be safe by the Food and Drug Administration or approved by the Environmental Protection Agency or Food Inspection Service of the United States Department of Agriculture.

The next two categories are related to and new to the Common Rule and introduce the concept of broad consent. Broad consent is an alternative consent process utilized only for the storage, maintenance, and secondary use of identifiable private information or identifiable biospecimens for future, yet-to-be-specified research.

For both exempt categories below, documentation of informed consent (i.e., broad consent) is required using an IRB-approved written form where the participant or legally authorized representative signs it and a copy of the informed consent form is provided to the person signing the form.

Storage or Maintenance for Secondary Research for Which Broad Consent is Required

In this category, the IRB must conduct a limited review to ensure that the investigator/sponsor has an effective process to track and retrieve identifiable biospecimens (i.e., chain of custody) and protect the privacy and confidentiality of identifiable private information maintained and stored as part of the collection of the data and biospecimens.

Secondary Research for Which Broad Consent is Required

In this category, the IRB must review the broad consent form and procedures for compliance with regulatory requirements for informed consent, including obtaining and documenting informed consent or a waiver of documentation of consent. Additionally, as part of broad consent, the investigator does not intend to return individual results from the research to participants as part of the investigational plan.

The use of broad consent has presented challenges to investigators and IRBs regarding implementation and oversight, respectively, for identifiable biospecimens and their chain of custody. The biospecimens are collected by the investigator but may not be stored or maintained by the investigator. The identifiable biospecimens may remain in the investigator's custody throughout the clinical investigation's lifecycle and after the trial is completed. The challenge is to track, retrieve, and destroy the identifiable biospecimens in the event the participant withdraws consent to use the biospecimens for future research. The investigator must show the IRB that there is a compliant process to achieve these and that the identifiable private information is protected to prevent unauthorized use and disclosure.

21 REVIEW OF RESEARCH

21 CFR Part 56.109 IRB Review of Research

a. *An IRB shall review and have authority to approve, require modifications in (to secure approval), or disapprove all research activities covered by these regulations.*
b. *An IRB shall require that information given to subjects as part of informed consent is in accordance with § 50.25. The IRB may require that information, in addition to that specifically mentioned in § 50.25, be given to the subjects when in the IRB's judgment the information would meaningfully add to the protection of the rights and welfare of subjects.*
c. *An IRB shall require documentation of informed consent in accordance with § 50.27 of this chapter, except as follows:*
    1. *The IRB may, for some or all subjects, waive the requirement that the subject, or the subject's legally authorized representative, sign a written consent form if it finds that the research presents no more than minimal risk of harm to subjects and involves no procedures for which written consent is normally required outside the research context; or*

2. *The IRB may, for some or all subjects, find that the requirements in § 50.24 of this chapter for an exception from informed consent for emergency research are met.*

d. *In cases where the documentation requirement is waived under paragraph (c)(1) of this section, the IRB may require the investigator to provide subjects with a written statement regarding the research.*
e. *An IRB shall notify investigators and the institution in writing of its decision to approve or disapprove the proposed research activity, or of modifications required to secure IRB approval of the research activity. If the IRB decides to disapprove a research activity, it shall include in its written notification a statement of the reasons for its decision and give the investigator an opportunity to respond in person or in writing. For investigations involving an exception to informed consent under § 50.24 of this chapter, an IRB shall promptly notify in writing the investigator and the sponsor of the research when an IRB determines that it cannot approve the research because it does not meet the criteria in the exception provided under § 50.24(a) of this chapter or because of other relevant ethical concerns. The written notification shall include a statement of the reasons for the IRB's determination.*
f. *An IRB shall conduct a continuing review of research covered by these regulations at intervals appropriate to the degree of risk, but not less than once per year, and shall have authority to observe or have a third party observe the consent process and the research.*
g. *An IRB shall provide in writing to the sponsor of research involving an exception to informed consent under § 50.24 of this chapter a copy of information that has been publicly disclosed under § 50.24(a)(7)(ii) and (a)(7)(iii) of this chapter. The IRB shall provide this information to the sponsor promptly so that the sponsor is aware that such disclosure has occurred. Upon receipt, the sponsor shall provide copies of the information disclosed to FDA.*
h. *When some or all of the subjects in a study are children, an IRB must determine that the research study is in compliance with part 50, subpart D of this chapter, at the time of its initial review of the research. When some or all of the subjects in a study that was ongoing on April 30, 2001, are children, an IRB must conduct a review of the research to determine compliance with part 50, subpart D of this chapter, either at the time of continuing review or, at the discretion of the IRB, at an earlier date.*

Amendment Review

Investigators are responsible for providing any and all information that modifies the clinical investigational plan. This includes amendments to the clinical trial protocol, Investigator Brochures (for drugs, biologics, and/or devices), informed consent forms, participant-facing material such as surveys, diaries, questionnaires, marketing and recruitment materials, and any other written or recorded information meant to be provided to participants. It is recommended that changes to documents such as clinical trial protocol, Investigator Brochures, informed consent, and participant-facing materials be red-lined in the documents in addition to providing a summary of changes for each document, as appropriate, as part of the document or separately to allow timely review by the IRB. Changes in key trial personnel (e.g., investigators and any trial personnel responsible for the conduct and/or reporting of the trial) must be submitted to the IRB as an amendment. Translated documents must also be submitted as amendments to the original application. Finally, laboratory manual amendments, pharmacy manual amendments, or any amendment to the operational manual are not required to be submitted to the IRB for review.

The use of clinical trial amendments, informed consent form(s) amendments, and participant-facing materials in the conduct of the clinical investigation must be implemented as soon as IRB approval is received. For translated documents, once the IRB acknowledges receipt, the investigator may begin using them. For informed consent form(s), the IRB shall instruct the investigator as to which participants must be reconsented, and in cases where reconsenting is indicated, the participants must be reconsented at the next clinic visit, regardless of whether the visit is in person or remote.

Continuing Review

The use of clinical trial amendments, informed consent form(s) amendments, and participant-facing materials in the conduct of the clinical investigation must be implemented as soon as IRB approval is received. For translated documents, once the IRB acknowledges receipt, the investigator may begin using them. For informed consent form(s), the IRB shall instruct the investigator as to which participants must be reconsented, and in cases where reconsenting is indicated, the participants must be reconsented at the next clinic visit, regardless of whether the visit is in person or remote.

Reportable Event Review

Reportable events include adverse events, serious adverse events, unanticipated adverse device effects, suspected unanticipated serious adverse reactions, and clinical investigational plan violations, also referred to as protocol deviations.

Not all safety events are to be reported to the IRB of record at the time of discovery. For adverse events and serious adverse events, only those that are unexpected, either in occurrence or frequency, must be reported at the time of discovery. All other non-reportable safety events must be documented and provided to the IRB for review upon request.

It is important for the investigators to review the IRB's record policies and procedures regarding reportable and non-reportable events and the timelines for reporting. The regulations do not provide timelines for reporting, instead stating prompt reporting is required. OHRP guidance recommends reporting (i) unanticipated serious adverse events within 1 week (7 calendar days) of the investigator becoming aware of the problem; and (ii) unanticipated problems (adverse events, violations) within 2 weeks (14 calendar days) of the investigator becoming aware of the problem. Many IRBs have adopted these timelines in their policies.

Close-Out and Completed Reviews

The status of clinical investigations must be shared with the IRB of record as an amendment as soon as the status changes. These include when the clinical investigation has completed enrollment and, therefore, it is closed to enrollment. Once all enrollment and all participants are off the study, the IRB will be informed that the clinical investigation is closed while data entry and review continue. Once all data has been entered by the investigator and reviewed by the sponsor for completeness, the clinical investigation is considered complete, and the IRB must be informed. Once a clinical investigation is completed, its IRB records are archived and available for inspection as needed. However, the clinical investigation is no longer overseen by the IRB, and no more submissions (i.e., continuing reviews, reportable events, amendments) are required or permitted.

IRB REVIEW DETERMINATIONS

21 CFR Part 56.113 Suspension or Termination of IRB Approval of Research

An IRB shall have authority to suspend or terminate approval of research that is not being conducted in accordance with the IRB's requirements or that has been associated with unexpected serious harm to subjects. Any suspension or termination of approval shall include a statement of the reasons for the IRB's action and shall be reported promptly to the investigator, appropriate institutional officials, and the Food and Drug Administration.

Investigators are encouraged to review the IRB record policies and procedures to better understand their determinations. Examples of common IRB determinations are listed below:

Approved – The investigator may move forward with opening the trial for participant enrollment utilizing the approved documents, including the stamped informed consent document(s).

Not Approved – The clinical investigation is not approved by the IRB, either during a full board meeting or Disapproval of clinical investigations subject to expedited, limited, or exempt review is not permitted. Disapproval recommendations from clinical investigations must be brought for discussion and adjudication during a full board meeting. The IRB must provide in writing the reasons for not approving the research, which the investigator may use to update the clinical investigational plan and documents for re-submission. In this case, the deficiencies are major and require significant revisions and submission as a new application.

Suspended – The IRB may suspend clinical investigation/research at any point during the clinical trial lifecycle for identified issues with participant safety and welfare as well as regulatory reasons, e.g., failure to submit a continuing review report, failure to submit reportable events, failure to follow IRB policies and procedures, and/or applicable regulations. The IRB must provide in writing the reasons for suspension. The suspension may be lifted by the IRB once the investigator complies with the specified non-compliance.

Terminated – The IRB may terminate clinical research/trial at any point due to non-compliance with IRB policies, procedures, and/or applicable laws and regulations. The IRB must provide in writing the reasons for termination. The investigator may appeal the decision. The IRB of record must have a written procedure for appeals.

Approved with Conditions – The investigator must fulfill the conditions provided by the IRB prior to opening the trial for enrollment. The IRB must provide the conditions in writing. This decision does not necessarily involve editing the clinical investigation documents, but instead possibly taking procedural steps to ensure compliance with applicable laws and regulations.

Modification Required – The investigator must make the requested modifications before the trial is approved. In this case, the IRB is requesting in writing amendments to some/all clinical investigation documents, including but not limited to informed consent, trial protocol, and other participant-facing documents/information.

Deferred – The application may be missing required information that prevents the IRB from reviewing it. IRB may request information/documents for the clinical investigational plan in writing that may require the application to come back to the full board for a re-review at a future meeting.

Acknowledged – This determination is reserved for the submission of reportable events and amendment documents other than trial protocol and/or participant-facing materials which do not require full board review.

Tabled without Action – In this instance, the clinical investigation is not reviewed by the IRB Full Board. In some cases, it is due to a request by the investigator to hold off on the review for a variety of reasons.

IRB RECORDS

21 CFR Part 56.115 IRB Records

a. *An institution, or where appropriate, an IRB, shall prepare and maintain adequate documentation of IRB activities, including the following:*
   1. *Copies of all research proposals reviewed, scientific evaluations, if any, that accompany the proposals, approved sample consent documents, progress reports submitted by investigators, and reports of injuries to subjects.*
   2. *Minutes of IRB meetings which shall be in sufficient detail to show attendance at the meetings; actions taken by the IRB; the vote on these actions including the number of members voting for, against, and abstaining; the basis for requiring changes in or disapproving research; and a written summary of the discussion of controverted issues and their resolution.*
   3. *Records of continuing review activities.*
   4. *Copies of all correspondence between the IRB and the investigators.*
   5. *A list of IRB members identified by name; earned degrees; representative capacity; indications of experience such as board certifications, licenses, etc., sufficient to describe each member's chief anticipated*

contributions to IRB deliberations; and any employment or other relationship between each member and the institution; for example: full-time employee, part-time employee, a member of governing panel or board, stockholder, paid or unpaid consultant.

6. *Written procedures for the IRB as required by § 56.108 (a) and (b).*
7. *Statements of significant new findings provided to subjects, as required by § 50.25.*

b. *The records required by this regulation shall be retained for at least 3 years after completion of the research, and the records shall be accessible for inspection and copying by authorized representatives of the Food and Drug Administration at reasonable times and in a reasonable manner.*

c. *The Food and Drug Administration may refuse to consider a clinical investigation in support of an application for a research or marketing permit if the institution or the IRB that reviewed the investigation refuses to allow an inspection under this section.*

IRBs are required to maintain adequate documentation of their activities. These include:

- Copies of all research applications submitted and reviewed and scientific evaluations, if any (e.g., Ancillary Committee Reviews and Determinations)
- Approved sample consent documents and participant-facing materials
- Continuing and progress reports submitted by investigators
- Reports of injuries to participants submitted by investigators
- Safety reports (e.g., adverse events, serious adverse events, unanticipated device effects, etc.) submitted by investigators
- Clinical trial protocol violation reports submitted by investigators
- Minutes of IRB meetings which shall be sufficiently detailed to show attendance, actions taken by the IRB, voting on these actions (including voting for, against and abstaining), basis for requiring changes to the research, disapproving research, and a written summary of the discussion of controverted issues and their resolution
- Documentation of continuing review activities, whether expedited or as part of a fully convened IRB meeting
  - Including rationale for conducting continuing reviews of clinical investigations that would not require continuing review.
- Copies of all correspondence between the IRB and the investigators.
  - Most IRBs utilize electronic platforms designed specifically to capture IRB activities. These platforms capture documentation of all IRB activities, including investigator applications, IRB administrator/coordinator initial reviews, minutes, and IRB-investigator communications. It is strongly recommended that investigators only communicate with the IRB through these platforms and not by regular electronic mail.
- List of all IRB members identified by name, earned degrees, representative capacity, and indications of experience such as board certifications, licenses, etc. The information listed for each member should be sufficient to describe each member's chief anticipated contributions to IRB deliberations.

Additionally, the list should include the member's employment or other relationship between the member and the institution. Each IRB should have financial disclosures for each member in order to assess any potential conflicts of interest that may affect deliberations.
- Written policies and procedures for the IRB
- Statements of significant new findings provided by participants

In the USA, IRB records must be retained for each clinical investigation or research project for at least 3 years after the completion of the clinical investigation/research project. Inactive records may be archived but must be accessible for inspection and copying by authorized representatives from applicable regulatory agencies. The electronic IRB platforms can store documentation indefinitely and assure compliance with record keeping regulations.

IRB REGULATIONS AND GUIDELINES

Before January 19, 2019, Food and Drug Administration (FDA – 21 CFR Parts 50 and 56) regulations and Department of Health & Human Services (DHS – 45 CFR Part 46 Subpart A [Revised Common Rule]) regulations regarding human participant protection and IRB were harmonized. Thereafter, the regulations have differed in some of their requirements.

IRB membership, responsibilities, and record-keeping have not changed, but there have been changes to the types of reviews based on the elements of consent to be discussed in Informed Consent Chapter and a Limited Review category that has been added by the Revised Common Rule.

ICH-E6(R2) follows the key IRB regulatory requirements of both 21 CFR Parts 50 and 56, and 45 CFR Part 46 Subpart A. On May 2023, ICH-E6(R3) draft was published for public comment. There are no significant updates regarding IRB responsibilities, composition, function, operations, procedures, or records in ICH-E6(R3) compared to ICH-E6(R2).

The main question is what regulatory requirements must IRBs follow now that the Federal IRB regulations are non-congruent. If the investigation is funded by a Federal agency or department, the IRB must comply with Revised Common Rule. If the investigation is overseen by the FDA, then the IRB must follow CFR Part 56. In some instances, both regulations apply, which investigators may find challenging to comply with. In other instances, neither regulation applies. In the latter case, many clinical investigations may fall under one of the exempt categories of the Revised Common Rule, and the IRB of record shall review accordingly.

The FDA has stated that it intends to harmonize its current regulations (21 CFR Parts 50 and 56) with the Revised Common Rule. In the meantime, the FDA has provided guidance (Impact of Certain Provisions of the Revised Common Rule on FDA-Regulated Clinical Investigations, October 2018) addressing their current stance on complying with the two regulations when both apply: *"Where the regulations differ, the regulations that offer greater protection to human subjects must be followed."* Given that the Revised Common Rule is more comprehensive, most IRBs are choosing to follow 45 CFR Part 46. It is important, however, for the investigator to review IRB policies and procedures prior to the submission of applications for review. IRB policies shall comply with all the applicable laws and regulations for their operation.

REGULATION OF IRBs

The IRB is an autonomous committee governed by policies and procedures designed to be compliant with applicable laws and regulations to protect participants' safety, welfare, and rights. IRBs are regulated by the FDA, OHRP, and DHHS and may be inspected at any time for compliance with applicable regulations. Clinical investigations overseen by the FDA (i.e., drugs and biologics under an IND, devices under an IDE) are subject to 21 CFR Part 56 regulatory requirements. Clinical investigations funded by or under the oversight of federal agencies or departments are subject to 45 CFR Part 46.

Further reading: FDA Institutional Review Boards Frequently Asked Questions, Guidance for Institutional Review Boards and Clinical Investigators, January 1998. https://www.fda.gov/regulatory-information/search-fda-guidance-documents/institutional-review-boards-frequently-asked-questions

9 Protected Health Information and Privacy in Clinical Trials

Sandra "Sam" Sather

INTRODUCTION

**This section does not include all requirements of HIPAA or all information about HIPAA and clinical research. This content is not intended to provide specific legal advice.*

The Health Insurance Portability and Accountability Act of 1996 (HIPAA) (Public Law 104-191) is a large set of regulations within the US healthcare system, enforced by the Office for Civil Rights (OCR), that applies to all covered entities (CE) (see Section "Covered Entity (CE)"). HIPAA aims to protect patient privacy and reinforce the security of patients' protected health information (PHI), especially as technological evolution continues to push healthcare into the online realm. HIPAA works in unison with International Council for Harmonization of Technical Requirements for Pharmaceuticals for Human Use (ICH) Good Clinical Practice (GCP) regulations and guidelines to ensure patients' privacy and safety while incorporating other Food and Drug Administration (FDA) regulations such as 21 CFR part 11, which pertains to the use of electronic records and signatures.[1] In 2023, both the FDA and the European Medicine Agency (EMA), in association with the ICH published guidelines for the use of electronic/computerized systems (eSystem) in clinical trials. The FDA's Electronic Systems, Electronic Records, and Electronic Signatures in Clinical Investigations: Questions and Answers and the EMA's Good Clinical Practice Inspectors Working Group (GCP IWG) Guideline on Computerized Systems and Electronic Data in Clinical Trials both advocate for the use of eSystems.[2,3]

Title II of HIPAA "Preventing Healthcare Fraud and Abuse; Administrative Simplification; Medical Liability Reform" includes the Administrative Simplification provision, which requires that the Department of Health and Human Services (HSS) define and adopt standards for dealing with electronically transmitted health information.[4] As a result, the HSS published "Standards for Privacy of Individually Identifiable Health Information", commonly referred to as the Privacy Rule, which defines appropriate use, electronic exchange, and disclosure of PHI.[5] This is highly relevant in clinical trials because while it is important to safeguard patients' PHI in a trial, it is equally important that the proper site personnel overseeing the safety of the patients and the sponsor monitoring personnel have access to these PHI. The Privacy Rule was not intended to burden clinical research; rather, it was intended

 DOI: 10.1201/9781003407010-9

to ensure that only the personnel whose roles required access to PHI, to complete data review for the study and/or uphold the patients wellbeing, are granted access to the PHI. The Privacy Rule also allows for CEs to compound the Informed Consent Forms with HIPAA authorization, which grants access to the individual's PHI to the CE for research purposes.

Following the Privacy Rule, the Security Rule was added to HIPAA under the Administrative Simplification Regulations in 2003, despite being proposed in 1998. The Security Rule established standards for safeguarding electronic PHI, including but not limited to changes to administrative, technical, and physical procedures.[6] The requirements of the Security Rule ensure that the confidentiality, integrity, and general access to electronic PHI remain protected. In order for both the Privacy and Security Rules to be enforced, the Enforcement Rule was proposed in 2005 and implemented in 2006.[7] This gave HHS the ability to investigate sites that were reported to not be in compliance with the Administrative Simplification Rules and, if deemed guilty of non-compliance, could be penalized with civil money fines. The final major amendment made to HIPAA was the final Omnibus rule, which sought to fill in any gaps or gray areas regarding the Administrative Simplification Rules and help streamline access to PHI in clinical trials. It also implemented provisions that came up through the Health Information Technology for Economic and Clinical Health Act (HITECH), which incentivized organizations to amend their protocols to have "meaningful use" of electronic health records (EHR).[8] This, in turn, would strengthen the Privacy and Security Rules by further refining the definition of permissible uses and disclosures of PHI.

Since the COVID-19 pandemic, there has been a need for decentralized clinical trials, telehealth visits, and electronic data capture to allow for continued participation in clinical trials. However, with these changes in how clinical trials are conducted, there is an increased risk of a security breach. HIPAA regulations play an integral part in facilitating this switch to these new technologies while supporting the security and integrity of the data in any media, along with additional FDA guidance on conducting clinical trials with the use of telehealth and HIPAA during and after the pandemic. HIPAA has been updated multiple times to include concepts such as enforcement and noncompliance consequences, civil penalties, unauthorized disclosures, expanded responsibilities of business associates, and CE responsibilities, especially in regards to compound and future authorizations. The following will further expand on these and other principles and concepts of HIPAA as they pertain to clinical trials.

HIPAA KEY TERMINOLOGY AND CORE CONCEPTS OF HIPAA IN CLINICAL TRIALS

Covered Entity (CE)

Covered entities are the stakeholders that must be compliant with the HIPAA regulations. CEs fall into one of three categories: health plans, healthcare clearinghouse, and health care providers (individuals, hospitals, or clinics), that send PHI electronically in connection with specific transactions defined in the HIPAA Privacy Rule.[9] These transactions include the following: health care claims (or equivalent encounter information), payments, or remittance advice, health care claims status, enrollment and disenrollment in a health plan, eligibility for a health plan, health plan premium payments, referral certification and authorization, final report of injury, health claim attachments, and regulation-prescribed transactions. If the entity falls into one or more of these categories, they are deemed covered in regards to HIPAA and are bound by the Privacy Rule.

Individual health care workers may fall into multiple CE categories, depending on the circumstances. If they are employees of a CE institution like a hospital, then they are considered part of that CE's workforce and are bound by their privacy policies and procedures, but they themselves are not considered CEs. However, if the health care worker operates a private practice, for example, an attending physician not employed by the hospital, and bills (or engages a third party to bill) electronically, they themselves are considered the CE. In this scenario, said physician is responsible for all the health information they create and maintain in their private practice, as opposed to delegating the task to the CE they worked out of. To be considered a CE, the individual or institution would need to perform covered functions that include treatment, payment, and any administrative activity that is considered a "health care operation". These covered functions are commonly referred to as TPOs. If an individual or institution does not perform TPO in relation to health information, they are not a CE and thus not required to follow HIPAA. Researchers that do not perform TPO activities as part of their research are not considered CEs and are not bound as individuals to the Privacy Rule. Research sites that do not provide managed care may not be CEs. For example, if a study participant needs medical care outside of the scope of the protocol during a trial, the non-CE would not treat the individual and invoice for their services; the study participant would need to go elsewhere for care.

Some institutions (e.g. academic medical centers) are considered hybrid entities because they have a mix of functions that would qualify them as CEs and functions that do not. In cases like this, the hybrid entities must define the functions that are covered by HIPAA and how the institution plans on upholding the corresponding requirements (e.g. HIPAA Authorization). Again, institutions that do not perform managed health care (e.g. providing medical care for treatment that is billed to the subject or using or disclosing PHI) are not considered CEs and therefore are not bound by the Privacy Rule. A university's independent research department would be an example, so long as there is no affiliation with any hospitals or medical schools and all subjects are recruited from outside a specific medical practice.

Protected Health Information (PHI)

The criteria for something to be considered "Health Information" recorded or oral in any form/medium are as follows: (i) is created or received by a health care provider, health plan, public health authority, employer, life insurer, school/university, or health care clearinghouse; and (ii) relates to the past, present, or future physical or mental health/condition of an individual. The Privacy Rule defines Protected Health Information (PHI) as individually identifiable health information transmitted or maintained in any form/medium. Two exceptions for PHI are education records covered by the Family Educational Rights and Privacy Act and employment records held by a CE in its role as an employer.

Written and Electronic HIPAA Authorization for Use/Disclosure of PHI

CEs must obtain a trial subject's written authorization (either the participants or their legal representative) to use or disclose any of their PHI that is not for treatment, payment, or healthcare operations unless permitted or required by the Privacy Rule.[10] HIPAA Authorization may also be done electronically, provided it is a "valid electronic signature" according to the Electronic Signatures in Global and National Commerce Act (ESign Act) (Public Law 106–229). If the ESign Act determines that an eSignature is valid, then all the legal effects of the signature are binding. The Privacy Rule also requires the CE to provide the subject (or legal representative) with a copy of the signed authorization regardless of whether it was written or electronic. A CE may rely on a third party to develop an authorization, like a research sponsor or ethics committee, but the CE has ultimate responsibility for compliance with the requirements of the content.

Research Use/Disclosure with Individuals' Authorization

CEs are permitted by the Privacy Rule to use and disclose PHI for research purposes with the research participant's authorization, which is presently sought out for most clinical trials and some records research. A valid authorization must satisfy the requirements of 45 CFR 164.508 "Uses and disclosures for which an authorization is required", in order for the CE to proceed with use/disclosure of PHI. Documentation of IRB or Privacy Board approval of a HIPAA Authorization is not required to use/disclose PHI.

The Privacy Rule contains Authorization requirements that apply to all uses/disclosure including research; however, there are several provisions that apply specifically to research authorization: (i) Unlike other authorizations, those for research purposes may state that the authorization does not expire, that there is no expiry date/event, or that the authorization continues until the "end of the research study". (ii) Authorization for use/disclosure of PHI may be combined with the Informed Consent Form to participate in the study or with any other legal permission related to the research study. (iii) An authorization for the use/disclosure of PHI for a research study may also be combined with an authorization for a different research activity. If research-related treatment is conditioned on the provision of one of the authorizations, then the compound authorization must clearly outline the conditional and unconditional in terms the patient can understand to be able to provide a proper authorization. The patient in this case must be presented with an opportunity to opt in or out of the unconditioned research activity. (iv) Authorization can be given for future research purposes if the form clearly outlines what that future research is as well as the patient's right to revoke their authorization.

Revoked Authorization

The Privacy Rule requires that for an authorization to be valid, it must contain, in plain language, specifics on the PHI being used/disclosed, who will have access to the PHI, the expiration date of the authorization, and the right to revoke their authorization in writing. If the patient does revoke their authorization, CEs may still use/disclose the patient's PHI for quality, safety, or effectiveness of FDA-regulated products' purposes pursuant to 45 CFR 164.508 and 45 CFR 164.512(b) (whether or not authorization is required). As permitted by these CFRs, the sponsor may also keep and review the collected data of the revoking patient as well as any other unmonitored information up until the date of the patient's revocation (unless stated otherwise in the CTA). In the event a patient withdraws their consent to the study (which can be done orally or written), it is required by the Privacy Rule that authorization properly inform the patient of their right to revoke their authorization, how they can revoke it (which can only be revoked via writing), and what exceptions there may be to the revocation. However, the Privacy Law does not require the researchers to suggest or request that a patient revoke their authorization to PHI after withdrawing their consent. It may be to the benefit of the researcher that the patient does not revoke their authorization since the researcher can then still use the data collected from the patient as long as it complies with 45 CFR 164.508 and 45 CFR 164.512(b).

Review Preparatory to Research (RPR)

Review Preparatory to Research (RPR) is a provision of the HIPAA Privacy Rule that allows researchers to use/disclose PHI for the single purpose of preparatory research without the patient's authorization, the option to agree or object, or an IRB approval of a waiver of authorization. This may be done, for example, to recruit prospective patients into a clinical study so long as the CE receives oral or written certification from the researcher that (i) the use/disclosure of the PHI is solely for research preparation, (ii) the researcher will not remove any PHI from the CE, and (iii) the sought PHI is necessary for research preparation. All three certifications are required to satisfy the 45 CFR 164.512(i)(1)(ii) provision. Under these provisions, CEs also have the option of allowing remote access to the PHI as long as those who access the PHI are bound to the three certifications and that the data is effectively safeguarded to OCR standards.[11]

De-identified Protected Health Information

Health information that is "de-identified" has had all of the features that may be used to identify an individual or provide any sort of reasonable basis for identity removed. This means the removal of all specific identifiers of an individual, their family, housemates, or employer. There are two options for obtaining de-identified information to meet the Privacy Rule's standard. The first and most direct and reliable would be to seek the help of an expert in the field. Through the use of statistical analysis and commonly used scientific principles, these experts can determine when PHI has a "very small risk" of being identifiable to an individual with any other generally available information. HSS has not yet defined what constitutes as a "very small risk", so it is generally in the opinion of the expert, and thus CEs should be cautious when entrusting de-identifying to an expert and review the information themselves before declaring it "de-identified". The second option for obtaining de-identified PHI is known as the "Safe Harbor" method, which is to strip the PHI of the 18 identifiers listed in 45 CFR 164.514(b)(2) and assure that the CE or any researcher has no additional information that, paired with the stripped PHI, could identify an individual. Certain codes may be retained in the de-identified PHI, assuming the code was not derived from another identifier and cannot be translated or used for another purpose.[12] Redacting study participant information practices common in clinical trials for things like safety reporting or remote monitoring are not as stringent as de-identification under HIPAA. The information for research must remain attributable to the study participant, like initials, but later would make the information not attributable to the study participant and therefore not usable for the trial. So the interchangeability between redaction and de-identification under HIPAA should be avoided.

Business Associate (BA)

CEs, especially health care providers and health plans, often delegate health care functions or transactions that involve the use/disclosure of PHI to third-party individuals or organizations, which are referred to as 'business associates" (BA).[13] These functions and transactions include those listed above (Section "Covered Entity (CE)") as well as administrative, accounting, actuarial, accreditation, legal, management, and any other function or transaction described in the Privacy Rule. In order to ensure that the BA follows the same rules and regulations, regarding the use/disclosure of PHI, as the CEs who gave the information, the Privacy Rule requires CE and BA relationships to be bound with a "business associate agreement".[14] The agreement should detail the limitations and obligations BAs have with the PHI as well as the consequences that would follow any breach to the agreement.

Clinical trial researchers and sponsors are not considered BAs since research is not a function that falls under the Privacy Rule's jurisdiction despite having access to the CEs PHI, however, researchers can be considered BAs if they were hired to create de-identified data or limited data sets for the CE. It is common practice for CEs participating in research to have researchers and sponsors enter clinical trial agreements (CTA) or data use agreements, similar to BA agreements, to ensure that everyone receiving the PHI will uphold its privacy and only use it for purposes outlined in the agreement. Confidential disclosure agreements (CDA) are another option CEs have to safeguard privacy. CDAs are often given to sponsor/contract research organization (CRO) representatives, such as monitors or clinical research associates (CRA), as an institutional requirement in order for them to access the PHI for a specific study. This practice has created challenges, since there is already a trial agreement in place between the sponsor and research site that includes confidentiality and agreed-upon language.

Requirements for Business Associates under the HITECH Rule

With the implementation of the HITECH Rule, BAs are now defined as any entity that creates, maintains, receives, or transmits data on behalf of the CE, with the sole exception of data transmission services. In addition, all the requirements of data privacy and security that applied to CEs now also apply to BAs, with similar penalties for breaches of these requirements, such as unauthorized disclosure. Penalties for noncompliance with BA can be up to $1.5 million, depending on the level of negligence observed. To avoid these penalties, BAs must maintain PHI protection and privacy to the sample level that is expected of CEs by applying reasonable and effective safeguards physically, technically, and administratively (e.g. routine security risk assessments). This applies to many services in clinical research that are either contracted or subcontracted as BAs of the CE, including recruiting, auditing, site operational consulting, and inspection preparation. A vendor of a BA, given they fit the definition of a BA, is also considered a BA and should be held to the same standards regarding data protection and privacy including entering into a business associate agreement. BAs are also now bound to both the Security Rule and certain aspects of the Privacy Rule, which include having written policies and SOPs, compliance with documentation requirements, conducting appropriate risk assessment and security training, evaluating security programs, and appointing a Security Officer. HSS has published a list of punishable violations of HIPAA for BAs on their website.[15] These include impermissible uses and disclosures of PHI, failure to comply with the security rule, failure to comply with the Minimum Necessary Standard (see Section "Minimum Necessary Standard (MNS)"), failure to provide accounting of disclosures when required, and more. Many of CE's business associate agreements and templates need to be updated in order to accommodate all of the added requirements of the HITECH Act.

Minimum Necessary Standard (MNS)

The Privacy Rule's primary objective is to keep PHI out of the hands of anyone who would use it to their own benefit or to the detriment of the patient. One way to combat this would be to try and limit the total amount of PHI that is shared without putting any hindrance on researchers accessing the data they need to complete the study. The Minimum Necessary Standard (MNS) is a component of the Privacy Rule that requires CEs and researchers to define what the absolute minimum amount of patients' PHI is required for their research goals.[5] Initially when this provision was put into place, it did hinder researchers to the extent that it is extremely difficult, in most cases, to define what that absolute minimum would be when developing research authorization for the use and disclosure of PHI. In response to the issue, the provision was modified so that once a patient gives a valid authorization to disclose their PHI, the researcher does not have to provide the necessary minimum. In other words, the MNS is exempt when an individual gives their authorization. For example, if a CE receives an individual's valid authorization to disclose their PHI to a sponsor/CRO, then the CE is not required to provide an MNS when disclosing any of the information listed on the authorization.

The MNS requires that CEs define what is an acceptable minimum for their organization and workforce, as this may vary depending on the industry. CEs may (but are not obligated to) rely on the researcher's request for PHI as meeting the MNS if it is accompanied by documentation from an IRB or Privacy Board that a waiver of authorization has been granted. CEs are also urged to constantly refine their procedures to cut out any unnecessary use or disclosure of PHI. Other exceptions to the MNS are disclosure to/request by a healthcare provider, if the person being disclosed to is the subject of the information or their legal representation, if the HSS is undergoing a complaint investigation, compliance review, or enforcement, if it is required by law, or if it is required for compliance with the HIPAA Transaction, Administrative Simplification, or other Rules. 45 CFR 164.502(a) is a list of allowed uses and disclosures of PHI under the Privacy Rule, such as disclosures for treatments, payments, and health care operations (TPO), as well as authorized purposes such as research.

Primary Care Physician's Right to Disclose PHI for the Purposes of Clinical Trial-Related Evaluation

Primary care providers (PCP) are a group whose disclosure of PHI to a research site is not covered by an authorization. Disclosure from a PCP of requested PHI is considered TPO, which is a permitted use of PHI according to 45 CFR 164.502(a) and does not need the patient's permission unless there are conflicting policies in place at the CE. The MNS does apply to the PHI disclosed by the PCP and should be recorded by the CE under their Privacy Practice. When the CE requests PHI from a PCP, the request should contain the specifics of what they consider to be the MNS for the study, why it is essential to the study, and the applicable timeframe under which the PHI will be used. From there, it is up to the PCP to assess the request and determine if the MNS is reasonable for its stated purpose in the request. When requesting PHI from a PCP, both the FDA and the Privacy Rule requirements must be met, which means that the requested PHI should have sufficient information so that investigators can be certain that no exclusionary criteria have been met and that the patient is eligible to participate in the study. Proper phrasing of an authorization is essential for its validity; according to 164.508(c)(1)(i), it must describe the use and disclosure of the PHI in a "specific and meaningful fashion" while still being valid under the Privacy Rule. Requesting an "entire medical record" or "complete patient file" is a valid authorization, whereas "all protected health information" goes beyond the MNS since all PHI would include items such as billing information, which is irrelevant in most clinical studies. It must also be written in a way that someone who has no understanding of PHI will comprehend what is being authorized when signing since most individuals reading the authorization will fall into that category.

Restriction of Source Data

Misinterpretation about the MNS has led some CEs to believe that they were the ones who determined how much PHI they disclosed to sponsors and monitors doing their reviews of the trials and, as a result, did not disclose the study pertinent medical records noted in the HIPAA Authorization that cover the protocol requirements for enrollment and study conduct and will be requested by the sponsors and monitors. If the amount of PHI the CEs disclose in this case is less than is referenced in the authorization, this may result in a failure to meet protocol and/or FDA requirements, and the associated penalties for this violation will apply. When an investigator is trying to obtain PHI for screening research subjects, it is essential they receive the PHI in order to comply with FDA requirements and to protect the safety of the potential trial subjects. Thus, CEs may use/disclose PHI to sponsors who are in an executed authorization, and sites should not restrict access to information for roles such as investigators provided that they are requesting PHI that is stated in the authorization.

Investigators are also required to have source documentation prepared for all patients in a study, including all protocol deviations, as well as observations and data that pertain to the study, which includes PHI such as nurses' notes or notes for the physician. In the event that each subject's case history is not provided, including their eligibility, adverse event assessments, and data integrity, then the subject's safety may be at risk. Sponsors and monitors are also required to review the PHI that is involved with a trial, and sites should not restrict access again, assuming that the PHI they are requesting is included in the authorization. To summarize, here is a quote from Jean Toth-Allen, Ph.D. from the FDA GCP program in an email about HIPAA and the disclosure of PHI to sponsors and monitors: "While HIPAA does have implications with regard to the conduct of clinical studies, HIPAA regulations do not interfere with or negate FDA regulations and our investigators do not look at any documents related to HIPAA requirements. Monitors for FDA-regulated studies are allowed access to subject records pertinent to the clinical study in question, and sponsors should report to the FDA when such refusals occur so the misconceptions of the hospital/institution in question can be corrected".

INFORMED CONSENT AND HIPAA AUTHORIZATION UNDER OMNIBUS RULEMAKING

The Omnibus Rule implemented many provisions of the Privacy Rule as a result of the HITECH Act, which sought to fill in any gaps or gray areas in the Privacy Rule and resolve any issues. One of these issues was the prohibition of compounding any PHI authorizations or informed consent forms, which meant that researchers and CEs had to seek multiple authorizations and consents for each individual research purpose, which led to more paperwork for administration to file and often confused the patients who had to read through each and every authorization and consent form. As mentioned above (Section "Research Use/Disclosure with Individuals' Authorization"), in March 2013, the HSS made an amendment to the Privacy Rule that allowed for CEs to combine authorizations with another conditioned or unconditioned authorization (e.g. informed consent). This amendment was meant to ease the burden on administration by not having multiple authorizations for every patient while simultaneously giving the patients less paperwork to try and understand before signing. A valid compound authorization must satisfy two criteria (see Section "Research Use/Disclosure with Individuals' Authorization" [iii]); (i) the conditioned and unconditioned components must be clearly defined, and (ii) there must be an opportunity for the individual to opt in/out of the unconditioned component of the authorization. CEs can add either an opt-in checkbox or a second signature for the unconditioned component, such as future research. The CE could also put an opt-in checkbox into the main authorization that specifically mentions the unconditioned component without a second signature.

When a patient revokes their authorization, unless they specify that they only wish to revoke a specific component of the authorization, the entire authorization stops and any PHI that is collected after the revocation can no longer be used or disclosed (see Section "Revoked Authorization"). HSS also made an amendment to the Privacy Rule regarding authorization for future unspecified studies. This was also meant to reduce the amount of paperwork required for administration and the patients by allowing CEs and researchers the option to add an authorization for future studies to the initial authorization. This amendment has similar criteria to compound authorizations: (i) there must be an adequate description of the intended future research and how the individual's PHI may be used or disclosed in it; and (ii) there must be an opt in/out choice given to each individual for the future research. All other requirements of the Privacy Rule on Authorizations still apply. The content of a compound authorization with informed consent can sometimes build up and make it hard for patients to fully understand the entire scope of what is being covered in the form. For this reason, some CEs and researchers will choose to separate the two documents for simplicity's sake.

Participant Privacy, Security, and Confidentiality When Utilizing Electronic Consent

Similar to paper consent forms, electronic informed consent (eIC) can be compounded with HIPAA authorization or kept separate at the CE's discretion. eICs used in US clinical trials under the FDA or OHRP should be able to ensure the confidentiality of the study participants identities, participation, and personal information and should not collect PHI unless authorization has been given by the participant. Compound documents often require more than one signature to account for the conditioned and unconditioned components of the document; depending on the technology used, there may not be an option for two signatures on one document. In this case, it is expected that the CE will either provide a paper copy of the compound document or separate it electronically into two documents, each with its own signature. It is also up to the CE to determine if one signature would suffice for a compound eIC and if the appropriate affirmations are linked to the signature, unless they choose to delegate the task to an ethics committee. HIPAA Privacy, Security, and Breach Notification Rules all apply the moment an eIC system of a CE or their BA begins to collect PHI, such as the requirement for data encryption.

SPONSOR RESPONSIBILITY TO MONITOR A SITE'S COMPLIANCE WITH THE PRIVACY RULE

A research sponsor has many duties that they need to be highly vigilant about to ensure that all the requirements of each regulatory body in a clinical trial (FDA, GCP, and OCR) are met. These duties and responsibilities are outlined in detail in 21 CFR 312.50-70. For example, all of the FDA requirements for a research site do not cover all the GCP requirements of the site. Unlike most FDA requirements, GCP requirements often involve state and local laws, depending on the study being conducted. In the case where a clinical trial has biohazardous waste on site, that site is also bound to OSHA rules and regulations regarding the safe handling and disposal of the waste. In a trial that deals with a controlled drug substance, the DEA's rules and regulations come into effect and it is the duty of the sponsor to ensure the site and its workforce are complying with these rules. HIPAA also has a set of rules and regulations that pertain specifically to CEs (see Section "Covered Entity (CE)") that are relevant to the quality performance of a research site. It is advised that sponsors determine which sites are CEs to understand what sites must be compliant with HIPAA before the trial begins. Sponsors must also routinely monitor the PHI being collected from trial participants before, during, and after a trial to satisfy 21 CFR 312.56 – "Review of ongoing investigations" as well as ensure the PHI is being used and disclosed in accordance with the Privacy Rule. Under the same CFR, a sponsor is required to ensure that the investigator (who is selected by the sponsor 21 CFR 312.50) is acting in compliance with the signed agreement (Form FDA-1572), the general investigational plan, and all the other requirements under 21 CFR 312.60 – "General responsibilities of Investigators".

Research sponsors, in most cases, are not CEs; they usually work with individuals or organizations that are CEs that are bound by the Privacy Rule (for more on CEs, see Section "Covered Entity (CE)" and for a list of CEs, see the HSS website[9]). Sponsors during site qualification should determine and document if the site is considered a CE and if so, what requirements they have for sponsor access to PHI. Remember, the CE is required to establish assurances that PHI is protected and has limited access when disclosed to non-CEs like sponsors. Part of this is because HIPAA notes that once the disclosure happens to a non-CE, it is no longer protected under the Privacy Rule. The OCR inspects CEs routinely and for cause. The sponsor could review a CE's history with OCR compliance reviews to see if they have had any past incursions with OCR and, if so, what remedial actions were taken. Finally, sponsors should not ask for unauthorized disclosures without a waiver from the individual or IRB. An example is the request for PHI of patients that have been pre-screened; this is pre-consent and authorization.

Additional Elements Commonly Requested by Sponsor under the Privacy Rule

Sponsors are required to monitor research and collect data to support marketing applications that involve the use and disclosure of PHI. They may also be required to blind members of the workforce as well as patients in order to comply with the study's design. In order to effectively satisfy these requirements, the sponsors will sometimes require additional elements in the HIPAA authorization. Some examples of elements include the following: (i) a statement that enrollment is conditional on the execution of an authorization. (ii) A statement describing the temporary suspension of the subject's rights to data review. The Privacy Rule permits a patient's right to access their PHI to be suspended while the trial is ongoing as long as the suspension is clearly explained in the authorization, including a designated timeframe for how long the suspension will last, and, of course, as long as the patient agrees and signs the authorization. (iii) The authorization should also clarify what PHI may be reviewed by the sponsor unless the authorization is revoked.

TELEHEALTH & HIPAA RELATED TO CLINICAL TRIALS

CEs are permitted under HIPAA to use remote communication technologies to provide telehealth services, so long as they do not violate any of HIPAA's Privacy, Security, or Breach Notification Rules.

The COVID-19 public health emergency forced most industries globally to either severely limit the amount of in-person work being done or halt it altogether. The clinical trial industry was no exception, with most medical sites being overrun with

COVID patients and barring entry to everyone not tending to the patients (nurses and doctors) on top of everyone (trial patients in this context) being told to remain in their homes. This meant that most trial participants could not go on-site for their scheduled visits, and therefore the only way for their participation to continue was through remote communications such as Telehealth. Since at the time many of these remote communications were novel concepts for most CEs, many would end up coming into conflict with HIPAA policies and regulations. The FDA published four "Notifications of Enforcement Discretion".[16] The "Enforcement Discretions" were concerning how Privacy, Security, Breach Notification, and Enforcement rules under HIPAA would be dealt with throughout COVID. Specifically, the fourth notification, "Notification of Enforcement Discretion for Telehealth Remote Communications During the COVID-19 Nationwide Public Health Emergency ("Telehealth Notification")", stated that noncompliance with certain HIPAA requirements would not be penalized if they were "in connection with the good faith provision of telehealth using a non-public-facing remote communication technology". This notification was intended to give support to CEs who, prior to COVID, had no experience with remote communications and may not have had policies and procedures in place to ensure their site's compliance with HIPAA's rules and regulations. Following a 90-day transition period, as of August 9th, 2023, the Enforcement Discretion expired, meaning that all violations of HIPAA's rules and regulations would be accordingly penalized. Post-COVID telehealth is still being used for managed care and for some clinical trial study visits. Research sites that are CEs are required to have procedures related to telehealth to safeguard the privacy and data security of their patients' PHI. HSS has guides, tips, and resources for using remote communications technologies for audio-only telehealth posted on their website for anyone seeking further information.[17–20]

SPONSOR REMOTE MONITORING OF SITES' PHI UNDER HIPAA

In 2013, the FDA and HHS released a guide called "Oversight of Clinical Investigations—A Risk-Based Approach to Monitoring" that outlines a sponsor's role in a clinical investigation as well as the rationale and methods behind "risk-based monitoring" in an effort to improve and ensure subject protection and study quality.[21] In the same year, in order to address the rising number of alternative methods for monitoring source data, especially remote access, the FDA and HHS also released another guide, "Electronic Source Data in Clinical Investigations", on how to effectively use electronic source data in a way that stays above FDA requirements.[22] Way before COVID, the HIPAA Privacy Rule does allow for CEs to grant remote access to PHI to researchers/sponsors for uses that qualify as reviews preparatory to research if that access is reasonable and appropriately safeguarded. The OCR published a guide on remote access to PHI in 2017 that provides further details,[11] which may be useful for sites and sponsors. However, reviews preparatory to research come before subject participation in a trial, so it does not apply to sponsor monitoring. On top of all the points covered in Section "Sponsor Responsibility to Monitor a Site's Compliance with the Privacy Rule" about sponsor responsibilities and duties when monitoring a site, sponsors may also complete many of their duties remotely, given that it does not conflict with any HIPAA requirements. This means that sponsors also need to do extra preparation when working with a site that allows remote access to source data.

Each CE can have different or more strict requirements. So sponsors must ensure their team members are aware of their assigned site requirements for remote review of any PHI. The following is a list of recommended processes sponsors should include when preparing to work at a site with remote access to source data: (i) Prepare a list of questions that will outline what data points are critical to the study and the timeline of the trial. Based on the answers, the sponsor must determine if having a remote option for source data will hinder the study or HIPAA compliance. (ii) Review all consent, agreement, and authorization documents to see if remote access to source data is clearly referenced. (iii) As a sponsor/CRO, make sure the CE's workforce is adequately educated and trained on the methods and systems you have chosen for remote monitoring and reviewing source data to promote compliance with all applicable requirements throughout the entire study's workforce. (iv) Conduct some form of interview/conversation with sites to determine the capability and expectations of working with sponsors/CRO monitors remotely. (v) Finally, outline a specified plan for remote monitoring and reviewing of source data and make sure that all personnel involved in the trial (CEs, researchers, investigators, Bas, etc.) are in some form of signed agreement.

CONCLUSION

HIPAA and all of its various rules and regulations cover primarily the security and privacy of health information in the US. In the context of clinical trials, HIPAA can be misunderstood to be a law that hinders the progress of clinical research due to the dozens of rules and regulations in place that define what can and what cannot be done with an individual's protected health information. On the contrary, many of the HIPAA amendments were in an effort to streamline access to this information while still upholding and enforcing the standards surrounding the security and privacy of PHI. Everyone involved in clinical trials (sponsors, covered entities, business associates, study participants etc.) should have a basic understanding of what HIPAA is and how it applies to their specific role in a clinical trial to ensure that they remain in compliance with the rules and regulations it enforces.

For further details on an individual's rights and responsibilities under HIPAA, visit the HHS website, which has numerous free guides and explanations of all the aspects of HIPAA, including FAQs. Additionally, OCR guides on HIPAA can be found on the HHS website, and the FDA also has published documents on HIPAA, which can be found on their own website as well.

REFERENCES

1. ICH. *ICH Harmonised Guideline - Good Clinical Practice (GCP) E6(R3).* International Council for Harmonization of Technical Requirements for Pharmaceuticals for Human Use. 19 May 2023. URL: https://database.ich.org/sites/default/files/ICH_E6%28R3%29_DraftGuideline_2023_0519.pdf.
2. FDA. *Electronic Systems, Electronic Records, and Electronic Signatures in Clinical Investigations Questions and Answers Guidance for Industry DRAFT GUIDANCE.* Food and Drug Administration. Revised 2023. URL: https://www.fda.gov/media/166215/download.

3. EMA. *Guideline on Computerised Systems and Electronic Data in Clinical Trials.* European Medicines Agency. 9 Mar 2023. URL: https://www.ema.europa.eu/en/documents/regulatory-procedural-guideline/guideline-computerised-systems-and-electronic-data-clinical-trials_en.pdf.
4. OCR. *HIPAA Administrative Simplification.* Department of Health and Human Services. Revised 26 Mar 2013. URL: https://www.hhs.gov/sites/default/files/hipaa-simplification-201303.pdf.
5. OCR. *OCR Privacy Brief - Summary of the HIPAA Privacy Rule - HIPPA Compliance Assistance.* Department of Health and Human Services. Revised May 2003. URL: https://www.hhs.gov/sites/default/files/privacysummary.pdf.
6. OCR. Security Rule. Department of Health and Human Services. Retrieved 29 Jan 2024. URL: https://www.hhs.gov/hipaa/for-professionals/security/index.html.
7. OCR. *The HIPAA Enforcement Rule. Department of Health and Human Services.* Retrieved 29 Jan 2024. URL: https://www.hhs.gov/hipaa/for-professionals/special-topics/enforcement-rule/index.html#:~:text=The%20HIPAA%20Enforcement%20Rule%20contains,Rules%2C%20and%20procedures%20for%20hearings.
8. OCR & HHS. *Modifications to the HIPAA Privacy, Security, Enforcement, and Breach Notification Rules under the Health Information Technology for Economic and Clinical Health Act and the Genetic Information Nondiscrimination Act; Other Modifications to the HIPAA Rules.* Federal Register. 25 Jan 2013. URL: https://www.govinfo.gov/content/pkg/FR-2013-01-25/pdf/2013-01073.pdf.
9. OCR. *Covered Entities and Business Associates.* Department of Health and Human Services. Retrieved 29 Jan 2024. URL: https://www.hhs.gov/hipaa/for-professionals/covered-entities/index.html.
10. FDA & HSS. *Guidance for Industry - IRB Review of Stand-Alone HIPAA Authorizations Under FDA Regulations.* Food and Drug Administration. 21 Oct 2003. URL: https://www.fda.gov/media/75279/download.
11. OCR. *21st Century Cures Act Guidance: Remote Access to PHI for Activities Preparatory to Research.* Department of Health and Human Services. Retrieved 29 Jan 2024. URL: https://www.hhs.gov/sites/default/files/remote-access-research-12-15-17.pdf.
12. OCR. *Guidance Regarding Methods for De-identification of Protected Health Information in Accordance with the Health Insurance Portability and Accountability Act (HIPAA) Privacy Rule.* Department of Health and Human Services. Retrieved 29 Jan 2024. URL: https://www.hhs.gov/hipaa/for-professionals/privacy/special-topics/de-identification/index.html.
13. OCR. *Business Associates.* Department of Health and Human Services. Retrieved 29 Jan 2024. URL: https://www.hhs.gov/hipaa/for-professionals/privacy/guidance/business-associates/index.html.
14. OCR. *Business Associate* Contracts. Department of Health and Human Services. Retrieved 29 Jan 2024. URL: https://www.hhs.gov/hipaa/for-professionals/covered-entities/sample-business-associate-agreement-provisions/index.html.
15. OCR. *Direct Liability of Business Associates. Department of Health and Human Services.* Retrieved 29 Jan 2024. URL: https://www.hhs.gov/hipaa/for-professionals/privacy/guidance/business-associates/factsheet/index.html.
16. HHS, OCR, & FDA. *Notice of Expiration of Certain Notifications of Enforcement Discretion Issued in Response to the COVID-19 Nationwide Public Health Emergency.* Federal Register. 13 Apr 2023. URL: https://public-inspection.federalregister.gov/2023-07824.pdf.
17. OCR. *HIPAA and Telehealth.* Department of Health and Human Services. Retrieved 29 Jan 2024. URL: https://www.hhs.gov/hipaa/for-professionals/special-topics/telehealth/index.html.

18. OCR. *Guidance on How the HIPAA Rules Permit Covered Health Care Providers and Health Plans to Use Remote Communication Technologies for Audio-Only Telehealth.* Department of Health and Human Services. Retrieved 29 Jan 2024. URL: https://www.hhs.gov/hipaa/for-professionals/privacy/guidance/hipaa-audio-telehealth/index.html.
19. OCR. *Telehealth Privacy and Security Tips for Patients.* Department of Health and Human Services. Retrieved 29 Jan 2024. URL: https://www.hhs.gov/hipaa/for-professionals/privacy/guidance/telehealth-privacy-security/index.html.
20. OCR. *Resource for Health Care Providers on Educating Patients about Privacy and Security Risks to Protected Health Information when Using Remote Communication Technologies for Telehealth.* Department of Health and Human Services. Retrieved 29 Jan 2024. URL: https://www.hhs.gov/hipaa/for-professionals/privacy/guidance/resource-health-care-providers-educating-patients/index.html.
21. FDA & HHS. *Guidance for Industry - Oversight of Clinical Investigations - A Risk-Based Approach to Monitoring.* Food and Drug Administration. Food and Drug Administration. Revised Aug 2013. URL: https://www.fda.gov/media/116754/download.
22. FDA & HHS. *Guidance for Industry - Electronic Source Data in Clinical Investigations.* Food and Drug Administration. Food and Drug Administration. Revised Sep 2013. URL: https://www.fda.gov/media/85183/download.

10 Good Pharmacovigilance Practices (GVP)

Jessica Chu

WHAT IS GVP AND WHAT IS PHARMACOVIGILANCE?

GVP stands for Good Pharmacovigilance Practices (GVP).

Pharmacovigilance, or PV for short, is generally described as:

- the study of the safety of marketed drugs under the practical conditions of clinical use in large communities (Ronald Mann, 2007);
- the science and activities relating to the detection, assessment, understanding and prevention of adverse effects or any other medicine-related problem (EMA, Pharmacovigilance: Overview, 2023); and
- the science and activities relating to the detection, assessment, understanding and prevention of adverse effects or any other medicine/vaccine-related problem (WHO, 2023b).

A BRIEF HISTORY OF PHARMACOVIGILANCE AND WHY IT IS IMPORTANT...

Pharmacovigilance, a science crucial for monitoring and ensuring the safe use of medications, has evolved in response to growing awareness of potential risks associated with drug use.

The history of pharmacovigilance can be traced back to the 1890s when fatalities were reported following increased chloroform use as an anaesthetic (Giulia Fornasier, 2018). A pivotal moment occurred between 1957 and 1962 when thalidomide, used by pregnant women to alleviate nausea in early pregnancy, led to severe adverse effects of congenital malformation in over 10,000 babies. The thalidomide tragedy highlighted the importance of monitoring the safety of medicinal products after marketing (Kim & Scialli, 2011). Thalidomide was withdrawn from marketing globally in 2006, but has been reintroduced with appropriate risk management activities for the treatment of a wide range of medical conditions such as leprosy, Crohn's disease, HIV, and also as a chemotherapeutic agent (Kim & Scialli, 2011; Vargesson, 2015; Waqas, Arfons, & Lazarus, 2011).

The thalidomide tragedy exposed safety limitations in drug development, emphasising issues in non-clinical and clinical trials, safety monitoring, limited samples size, participant selection bias, insufficient duration of follow-up of trial subjects, and limited follow-up post-trial (Kim & Scialli, 2011; Loke, 2012). It underscored

DOI: 10.1201/9781003407010-10

the necessity for continuous monitoring throughout a drug's lifecycle to assess long-term effects on the treatment population and emphasised the limitations of animal testing models.

How did National Medicine Regulatory Authorities Respond?

The thalidomide disaster led to the establishment of many of the drug regulatory mechanisms of today. These regulatory mechanisms mandate rigorous review and approval of all new applications for medicinal product licences by regulatory authorities before they become available for clinical use. For example, regulatory authorities introduced independent committees of advisors, medicines regulations, and drug surveillance systems to oversee the drug licensing and approval process. Notably, the United Kingdom (UK) government established the Committee on the Safety of Drugs (the Dunlop Committee) in June 1963 to provide advice regarding the quality, safety, and efficacy of medicines. This expert committee was further strengthened with the enactment of the Medicines Act of 1968, establishing the legal foundation for licensing medicinal products in the UK.

In 1964, the UK's Medicines and Healthcare Products Regulatory Agency (MHRA) established the Yellow Card reporting scheme to collect adverse drug reaction reports associated with the use of medicinal products. Over the years, this system has been expanded to include vaccines, herbal remedies, and other healthcare products. Not long after, the US Food and Drug Administration (FDA) implemented the Adverse Drug Reaction Reporting System (ADRRS) database in 1969, and following multiple redesigns and relaunches over the years, the system has transformed into the current safety reporting system known as the FDA Adverse Event Reporting System (FAERS) (Ahmad, 2003; NBER, 2023; Sonawane, Cheng, & Hansen, 2018). On a more global level, the World Health Organisation Uppsala Monitoring Centre (WHO-UMC) established the Programme for International Drug Monitoring (PIDM) to collect, investigate, and monitor adverse drug reactions to medicines. The WHO-UMC PIDM now has over 170 full and associated member countries, and therefore covers approximately 99% of the world's population (Uppsala Monitoring Centre, 2023).

The data gathered by these national and international systems for analysis plays a crucial role in identifying potential safety issues and assessing the safety of medicinal products post-market approval. There are other non-profit scientific organisations dedicated to promoting pharmacovigilance, and the safe and effective use of medicinal products such as the European Society of Pharmacovigilance (ESOP), which was founded in 1992. The ESOP transformed into the International Society of Pharmacovigilance (ISoP) in 2000, and continued its commitment to advancing global drug safety (International Society of Pharmacovigilance, 2023, April 11).

In the European Union (EU), the European Medicines Agency (EMA) was established in 1995 with the aim to harmonise the efforts of national regulatory authorities within the EU/European Economic Area (EEA) region. Key deliverables of the EU's legal framework for pharmacovigilance, outlined in Directive 2010/84/EU and Regulation (EU) No. 1235/2010 of the European Parliament and of the Council of 15 December 2010, were the EMA guidelines for Good Pharmacovigilance Practice

(GVP). These regulations were built upon earlier directives and regulations, namely, Directive 2001/83/EC and Regulation No. 726/2004.

The EU's pharmacovigilance legislation, complemented by Commission Implementing Regulation No. 520/2012, ensures operational details and expectations for the pharmacovigilance system. Amendments in October 2012, through Regulation (EU) No. 1027/2012 and Directive 2012/26/EU, aimed to enhance transparency and address safety issues across all EU Member States.

The EU GVP guidelines, designed to facilitate pharmacovigilance performance, apply to Marketing Authorisation Holders (MAH) (i.e., medicinal product license holders), the EMA and regulatory authorities in EU Member States. While initially intended for EU states and the EMA, these guidelines have been adopted by countries outside the EU, including EEA members and the UK. Covering medicines authorised centrally and nationally, the GVP guidelines consist of distinct chapters (referred to as the GVP Modules), each covering a key component of the PV system. Developed collaboratively by the EMA, national regulatory authorities, and industry experts, the modules are designed to be practical, adaptable to new developments, and responsive to emerging safety concerns, supporting harmonisation across the EU/EEA (EMA, Pharmacovigilance: Overview, 2023). An overview of the modules of the GVP guidance is provided in Table 10.1.

Pharmaceutical companies and stakeholders must remain vigilant and stay informed about changes in regulations and guidelines in the countries where they market their products. Compliance with these regulations is essential to ensure the acceptable quality, safety, and efficacy of medicinal products. Regulatory authorities may also opt to join the International Council for Harmonisation (ICH). The ICH serves as an initiative to harmonise pharmaceutical development and approval processes, fostering the creation of safe, effective, and high-quality medicines. This is achieved through the attainment of scientific consensus between regulatory authorities and the pharmaceutical industry within the participating ICH member countries. Comprising experts from regulatory bodies and the pharmaceutical industry worldwide, ICH members collaboratively address scientific and technical aspects of pharmaceuticals, resulting in the development of ICH guidelines covering safety, quality, efficacy, and various multidisciplinary topics (ICH, 2023) (Table 10.2).

THE EU GVP MODULES AND BEYOND

As mentioned previously, GVP is a set of guidelines developed to improve the quality of pharmacovigilance across the EU and the EEA and to ensure the protection of public health by detecting, assessing, understanding, and preventing adverse effects or any other drug-related problems (EMA, 2022). In general, each EU member state may follow the EMA GVP in its entirety or impose slightly different requirements for MAHs operating in its territory. It is therefore important to check the national requirements, especially for products authorised through purely national procedure or *via* the mutual recognition procedure.

Since the publication of the EU GVP guidelines, non-EU countries and regions around the world have implemented their own regulations and guidelines for pharmacovigilance with varying degrees of detail (and therefore interpretations).

Table 10.1
Overview of the Adopted European Guidelines on Good Pharmacovigilance Practices (GVP) Modules, Product- or Population-Specific Considerations, and Annexes

Title	Publication History (Effective Dates)
GVP Modules	
Introductory cover note, last updated with release of Addendum III of Module XVI	March 2022
Module I – Pharmacovigilance systems and their quality systems	July 2012
Module II – Pharmacovigilance system master file	July 2012
Revision 1	April 2013
Revision 2	March 2017
Module III – Pharmacovigilance inspections	December 2012
Revision 1	September 2014
Module IV – Pharmacovigilance audits	December 2012
Revision 1	August 2015
Module V – Risk management systems	July 2012
Revision 1	April 2014
Revision 2	March 2017
Module VI – Collection, management and submission of reports of suspected adverse reactions to medicinal products	July 2012 September 2014
Revision 1	November 2017
Revision 2	
Module VI Addendum I – Duplicate management of suspected adverse reaction reports	November 2017
Module VII – Periodic safety update report	July 2012
Revision 1	December 2013
Module VIII – Post-authorisation safety studies	July 2012
Revision 1	April 2013
Revision 2	August 2016
Revision 3	October 2017
Module VIII Addendum I – Requirements and recommendations for the submission of information on non-interventional post-authorisation safety studies	July 2012 April 2013 August 2016
Revision 1	June 2020
Revision 2	
Revision 3	
Module IX – Signal management	July 2012
Revision 1	November 2017
Module IX Addendum I – Methodological aspects of signal detection from spontaneous reports of suspected adverse reactions	November 2017
Module X – Additional monitoring	April 2013
Modules XI, XII, XIII, XIV – the planned topics have been addressed by the other Modules and Annexes.	Void

(Continued)

Table 10.1 (*Continued*)
Overview of the Adopted European Guidelines on Good Pharmacovigilance Practices (GVP) Modules, Product- or Population-Specific Considerations, and Annexes

Title	Publication History (Effective Dates)
GVP Modules	
Module XV – Safety communication	January 2013
Revision 1	October 2017
Module XVI – Risk minimisation measures: selection of tools and effectiveness indicators	March 2014 April 2014
Revision 1	March 2017
Revision 2	
Module XVI Addendum I – Educational materials	December 2015
Final GVP Product- or Population-Specific Considerations	
I: Vaccines for prophylaxis against infectious diseases	December 2013
II: Biological medicinal products	August 2016
Product- or Population-Specific Considerations III	Void
IV: Paediatric population	November 2018
Committee for Medicinal Products for Human Use (CHMP) Guideline on safety and efficacy follow-up – risk management of advanced therapy medicinal products	December 2008
Annex	
Annex I – Definitions	July 2012
Revision 1	December 2012
Revision 2	January 2014
Revision 3	April 2014
Revision 4	October 2017
Annex II – Templates: Cover page of Periodic Safety Update Report (PSUR)	July 2012
Revision 1	April 2013
Annex II – Templates: Direct Healthcare Professional Communication (DHPC)	January 2013
Revision 1	October 2017
Annex II – Templates: Communication Plan for Direct Healthcare Professional Communication (CP DHPC)	October 2017
Annex III – Guideline on the exposure to medicinal products during pregnancy: need for post-authorisation data	May 2006
Annex III – Note for guidance – EudraVigilance Human – Processing of safety messages and individual case safety reports (ICSRs)	October 2010
Annex III – Overview of comments received on draft note for guidance EudraVigilance version 7.1 processing of safety messages and individual case safety reports (ICSRs)	November 2009
Annex III – Draft note for guidance EudraVigilance human version 7.1 processing of safety messages and individual case safety reports (ICSRS)	April 2008

(*Continued*)

Table 10.1 (*Continued*)
Overview of the Adopted European Guidelines on Good Pharmacovigilance Practices (GVP) Modules, Product- or Population-Specific Considerations, and Annexes

Title	Publication History (Effective Dates)
GVP Modules	
Annex IV – International Conference on Harmonisation of Technical Requirements for Registration of Pharmaceuticals for Human Use (ICH) guidelines for pharmacovigilance	see Table 10.3
Annex V – Abbreviations	April 2013
Revision 1	October 2017
Pharmacovigilance Guidance and Publications that were Developed Outside of the EMA GVP Process	
• Pharmacovigilance: regulatory and procedural guidance • Guidance on the format of the risk management plan (RMP) in the EU – integrated format • Consideration on core requirements for RMPs of COVID-19 vaccines • Signal management • EudraVigilance • European Medicines Agency policy on access to EudraVigilance data for medicinal products for human use – Revision 3 • Union reference dates and submission of periodic safety update reports • Guideline on registry-based studies – Scientific guideline • Standards and guidances of the European Network of Centres for Pharmacoepidemiology and Pharmacovigilance (ENCePP) • Guideline on key aspects for the use of pharmacogenomics in the pharmacovigilance of medicinal products • Good practice guide on recording, coding, reporting and assessment of medication errors • Good practice guide on risk minimisation and prevention of medication errors • Risk minimisation strategy for high strength and fixed combination insulin products, developed as an addendum to the good practice guide on risk minimisation and prevention of medication errors	See publication

Source: https://www.ema.europa.eu/en/human-regulatory/post-authorisation/pharmacovigilance/good-pharmacovigilance-practices (accessed on 24 January 2024).

Currently, the European legislation and guidelines on pharmacovigilance stand out as the most comprehensive and user-friendly resources available for MAHs. Notably, several non-European countries such as the United Arab Emirates (UAE) and Turkey have closely aligned their pharmacovigilance requirements with those of Europe, making adjustments as needed. Similarly, the UK MHRA, which contributed to the EU pharmacovigilance guidelines, has continued to embrace European legislation post-Brexit, with certain exceptions outlined in the MHRA Guidance on Exceptions

Table 10.2
Overview of The International Council for Harmonisation of Technical Requirements for Pharmaceuticals for Human Use (ICH) Guidelines for Pharmacovigilance (GVP Annex IV)

ICH Topic https://www.ich.org/	Date of Step 4
E2A Clinical Safety Data Management: Definitions and Standards for Expedited Reporting	October 1994
E2B (R3) Clinical Safety Data Management: Data Elements for Transmission of Individual Case Safety Reports (ICSRs)	November 2012
E2B (R3) Q&As: Clinical Safety Data Management: Data Elements for Transmission of Individual Case Safety Reports	January 2023
E2C (R2) Periodic Benefit-Risk Evaluation Report	December 2012
E2C (R2) Q&As: Periodic Benefit-Risk Evaluation Report	March 2014
E2D Post-Approval Safety Data Management: Definitions and Standards for Expedited Reporting	November 2003
E2E Pharmacovigilance Planning	November 2004
E2F Development Safety Update Report	August 2010
M1 Medical Dictionary for Regulatory Activities (MedDRA) https://www.meddra.org/	January 1999
M2 Electronic Standards for the Transfer of Regulatory Information (ESTRI). It was decided that the M2 Expert Working Group (EWG) would no longer directly involved in the development of technical solutions in relations to topics such as E2B (R3) and M5 but would instead provide the framework for the efficient and effective development of the solutions by groups dedicated to these topics.	Void

Note: Date of implementation of Step 4 varies for different Regulatory Authorities. Refer to website for the Step 5 implementation status for the different ICH country members.

and Modifications to the EU Guidance on Good Pharmacovigilance Practices applicable to UK MAHs (MHRA 2020, December 21). Therefore, it is important to recognise the vast and complex regulatory landscape that MAHs must be familiar with to ensure compliance with the national pharmacovigilance requirements in the countries where they and/or their licensing partners operate. Since many MAHs tend to operate globally, they are faced with a wide and ever-changing regulatory landscape, which may pose additional challenges due to differences in regulatory terminology between different countries and regions.

Compliance with pharmacovigilance regulations is essential for ensuring that medicinal products are safe and effective and for maintaining public confidence in the pharmaceutical industry. GVP Module III 'Pharmacovigilance inspections' describes the possible regulatory actions against a marketing authorisation when non-compliance is detected. These actions include product recalls, warning letters, amendments to clinical trials due to product-specific safety issues and directed regulatory authority inspections. In cases of serious non-compliance, actions may include suspension or withdrawal of marketing authorisation(s), financial penalties, and/or referral for criminal prosecution with the possibility of imprisonment for individuals found responsible.

A non-exhaustive list of health authority resources (i.e., websites and links) for pharmacovigilance, including national and regional requirements, is presented in Table 10.3. This is to illustrate the vast amount of information available and the country requirements that need to be considered and followed to navigate the global regulatory landscape. It should be noted that there is also a varying degree of details between the regulatory authorities, and some information is only available in the national language.

Recent Examples of Pharmacovigilance in Action

Below are recent examples of pharmacovigilance in action in modern medicine to show its vital role in safeguarding public health throughout the lifecycle of a medicinal product. Other benefits to pharmacovigilance are that it can help reduce healthcare costs by reducing the number of adverse events and improving the efficiency of drug development and regulation. The application and benefit of pharmacovigilance to modern medicine is undeniable, and its importance is only increasing as we continue to rely on medications to improve and maintain our health.

COVID-19

Pharmacovigilance has played a key role in the COVID-19 pandemic in monitoring and analysing near real-time data pertaining to the safety of drugs and vaccines used in the treatment and prevention of COVID-19 (WHO, Global Convening on COVID-19 Vaccination Monitoring and Related System Strengthening, 2023a). The pandemic has sparked contentious discussions and heightened public interest regarding the safety of vaccines to an extent never seen before.

Pharmacovigilance systems were adeptly adjusted to address the unique challenges posed by the pandemic. This involved the imperative for real-time monitoring of an extensive volume of vaccine safety data, the implementation of swift reporting systems for side effects, and the identification of potential safety concerns before major issues arose (Sabine Jeck-Thole, 2023).

The situation also saw the collaboration and swift response by regulatory authorities and MAHs to ensure the COVID-19 vaccines could be made available to the public with tailored pharmacovigilance planning. In Europe, the regulatory authorities granted conditional marketing approval for several COVID-19 vaccines and implemented an accelerated evaluation process as well as the Pharmacovigilance Plan of the EU Regulatory Network for COVID-19 Vaccines (EMA, Pharmacovigilance Plan of the EU Regulatory Network for COVID-19 Vaccines, 2020). The Pharmacovigilance Plan outlined specific obligations for MAHs such as the submission of aggregate reports at a higher frequency (monthly intervals) instead of the standard submission frequency of six-monthly intervals in the first year of authorisation. The accelerated process also included collection of exposure data and conduct of post-authorisation safety studies (PASS) in a narrow time window. Furthermore, regulatory authorities and global organisations implemented ongoing surveillance, regularly issuing

Table 10.3
List of National Regulatory Authority Resources Relevant to Pharmacovigilance

Country	Regulatory Authority	Regulatory Authority Website[a]	PV Guidance and Related Links[a]
Australia	The Therapeutic Goods Administration (TGA)	https://www.tga.gov.au/	Pharmacovigilance responsibilities of medicine sponsors https://www.tga.gov.au/resources/resource/guidance/pharmacovigilance-responsibilities-medicine-sponsors
Brazil	Agência Nacional de Vigilância Sanitária – Anvisa (ANVISA)	https://www.gov.br/anvisa/pt-br/english	PV Bulletins and other publications https://www.gov.br/anvisa/pt-br/centraisdeconteudo/publicacoes/monitoramento/farmacovigilancia Regulatory Guide: http://antigo.anvisa.gov.br/documents/33868/2894051/Periodical_Pharmacovigilance_Report.pdf/ceee3b13-b2f6-48fe-ba3c-bf463c4c40b6?version=1.0
China	National Medical Products Administration (NMPA)	http://english.nmpa.gov.cn/	Good Pharmacovigilance Practice: http://english.nmpa.gov.cn/2021-05/13/c_655095.htm Drug Administration Law of the People's Republic of China: https://www.nmpa.gov.cn/xxgk/fgwj/flxzhfg/20190827083801685.html
Canada	Health Canada (HC)	https://www.canada.ca/en/health-canada.html	GVP Guidelines (GUI-0102) https://www.canada.ca/en/health-canada/services/drugs-health-products/compliance-enforcement/good-manufacturing-practices/guidance-documents/pharmacovigilance-guidelines-0102.html
European Union (EU)[b] and the European Economic Area (EEA)	European Medicines Agency (EMA)	https://www.ema.europa.eu/en	GVP Modules https://www.ema.europa.eu/en/human-regulatory/post-authorisation/pharmacovigilance/good-pharmacovigilance-practices

(Continued)

Table 10.3 (*Continued*)
List of National Regulatory Authority Resources Relevant to Pharmacovigilance

Country	Regulatory Authority	Regulatory Authority Website[a]	PV Guidance and Related Links[a]
Eurasian Economic Union (EAEU)[c]	EAEU Member States	EAEU detailed PV processes https://eec.eaeunion.org/en/news/v-eaes-detalizirovany-protsessy-farmakonadzora/	EAEU Economic Commission Council Resolution No. 78 https://docs.eaeunion.org/docs/en-us/01127650/cncd_21112016_doc.pdf
India	Central Drugs Standard Control Organization (CDSO)	CDSO https://cdsco.gov.in/opencms/opencms/en/Home/	PV Guidance Document for MAHs of Pharmaceutical Products https://ipc.gov.in/mandates/pvpi/publications/8-category-en/1222-guidance-documents.html
Israel	Israel Ministry of Health (Israel MoH)	https://www.gov.il/en/departments/ministry_of_health/govil-landing-page	Pharmacy Division – Risk Management and Drug Information Department https://www.gov.il/he/Departments/General/drug-risk-conf
Japan	The Ministry of Health, Labour and Welfare (MHLW), and	MHLW https://www.mhlw.go.jp/english/index.html	Pharmaceutical Administration and Regulations in Japan https://www.jpma.or.jp/english/about/parj/individual.html Post-marketing Safety Measures: https://www.pmda.go.jp/english/safety/info-services/0001.html
	Japanese Pharmaceuticals and Medical Devices Agency (PMDA)	PMDA https://www.pmda.go.jp/english/index.html	
Mexico	Comisión Federal para la Protección contra Riesgos Sanitarios (COFEPRIS)	https://www.gob.mx/cofepris/	Guides, Guidelines and PV Requirements: https://www.gob.mx/cofepris/documentos/guias-lineamientos-y-requerimientos-de-farmacovigilancia
New Zealand	New Zealand Medicines and Medical Devices Safety Authority (MedSafe)	https://www.medsafe.govt.nz/	Guideline on the Regulation of Therapeutic Products in New Zealand: https://www.medsafe.govt.nz/regulatory/guideline/grtpnz/part-8-pharmacovigilance.pdf

(*Continued*)

Table 10.3 (*Continued*)
List of National Regulatory Authority Resources Relevant to Pharmacovigilance

Country	Regulatory Authority	Regulatory Authority Website[a]	PV Guidance and Related Links[a]
Philippines	Philippines Food and Drug Administration (PFDA)	https://www.fda.gov.ph/	FDA Circular No. 2020-003, Guidelines for Pharmaceutical Industry on Pharmacovigilance https://www.fda.gov.ph/fda-circular-no-2020-003-guidelines-for-pharmaceutical-industry-on-pharmacovigilance/ PV information https://www.fda.gov.ph/pharmacovigilance/
South Africa	South African Health Products Regulatory Authority (SAHPRA)	www.sahpra.org.za	Medicines and Related Substances Act (previously Drugs Control Act) 101 of 1965 https://www.gov.za/documents/drugs-control-act-7-jul-1965-0000#:~:text=The%20Medicines%20and%20Related%20Substances,for%20matters%20incidental%20thereto
South Korea	Korea Ministry of Food and Drug Safety (MFDS)	https://www.mohw.go.kr/eng/	Regulation on Safety of Pharmaceuticals, etc. https://www.mfds.go.kr/eng/brd/m_18/view.do?seq=71527
Taiwan	Taiwan Food and Drug Administration (TFDA)	https://www.fda.gov.tw/eng/	Regulation for the Management of Drug Safety Surveillance https://www.fda.gov.tw/eng/lawContent.aspx?cid=5060&id=3156
Turkey	Türkiye İlaç ve Tıbbi Cihaz Kurumu (TITCK)	https://www.titck.gov.tr/	PV Guidelines for Registration Holders of Medicinal Products for Human Use https://titck.gov.tr/PortalAdmin/Uploads/UnitPageAttachment/QSI4TS8m.pdf

(*Continued*)

Table 10.3 (*Continued*)
List of National Regulatory Authority Resources Relevant to Pharmacovigilance

Country	Regulatory Authority	Regulatory Authority Website[a]	PV Guidance and Related Links[a]
United Kingdom	The Medicines and Healthcare products Regulatory Agency (MHRA)	https://www.gov.uk/government/organisations/medicines-and-healthcare-products-regulatory-agency	Guidance on PV procedures https://www.gov.uk/government/publications/guidance-on-pharmacovigilance-procedures/guidance-on-pharmacovigilance-procedures The Human Medicines Regulations 2012 https://www.legislation.gov.uk/uksi/2012/1916/contents/made From 1st January 2021, the MHRA became the UK's standalone medicines and medical devices regulator because of the withdrawal of the UK from the EU. Prior to this date EMA GVP Modules was in force and continued to be followed with exceptions and modifications to the EU guidance on GVP.
United States	The US Food and Drug Administration (US FDA)	https://www.fda.gov/drugs	Code of Federal Regulations. Title 21: Food and Drugs. Part 314: Applications for FDA Approval to Market a New Drug. Subpart D: Postmarketing Reporting of Adverse Drug Experiences https://www.ecfr.gov/current/title-21/chapter-I/subchapter-D/part-314#se21.5.314_110
United Arab Emirates	The UAE Ministry of Health and Prevention (UAE MoH)	https://mohap.gov.ae/en/home	Pharmacovigilance Dashboard https://www.doh.gov.ae/en/research/Dashboard/Pharmacovigilance GVP for MAHs/ Pharmaceutical Manufacturers in UAE https://mohap.gov.ae/assets/cd584ee8/UAE%20MOH%20GVP%20Guidlines%20ver%201.2.pdf.aspx

[a] The URL addresses provided in Table 10.3 were accessed on 24 January 2024.

[b] The EU member states: Austria, Belgium, Bulgaria, Croatia, Republic of Cyprus, Czech Republic, Denmark, Estonia, Finland, France, Germany, Greece, Hungary, Ireland, Italy, Latvia, Lithuania, Luxembourg, Malta, Netherlands, Poland, Portugal, Romania, Slovakia, Slovenia, Spain, and Sweden. The EEA member states: Iceland, Norway, and Liechtenstein

[c] The EAEU member states: Armenia, Belarus, Kazakhstan, Kirghizstan, and Russia

publications concerning the safety and potential side effects of COVID-19 vaccines, utilising data from their databases. This initiative enabled the public to access current, accurate, and reliable information regarding the safety of COVID-19 treatments and vaccines.

It is a requirement for MAHs to promptly update the product label, a document describing the properties, known safety information, and officially approved conditions of use for a medicine, in response to newly acquired information about the product.[1] New information could be gathered through routine pharmacovigilance activities such as the collection and analysis of safety information (adverse events, adverse drug reactions, and special situations). It must be highlighted that spontaneous reporting of adverse events may not have proven causal association and may not be medically confirmed to the suspect medicine. However, spontaneous reports from patients/consumers are by default considered related to the suspect drug/vaccine even without medical confirmation by a healthcare professional.

Notably some of the serious and uncommon adverse events experienced by people receiving the coronavirus vaccines in the US included myocarditis (inflammation of the heart muscle) and pericarditis (inflammation of the lining outside the heart) for the Pfizer-BioNTech (INN: tozinameran) or Moderna (INN: elasomeran) (Prevention, 2023). Several reports of blood clots (Thrombosis with thrombocytopenia syndrome, TTS) were reported following the administration of the Johnson & Johnson (Ad26. COV2-S) vaccine and reports of blood clotting disorders were associated the Oxford/ AstraZeneca (ChAdOx1 nCoV-19) vaccine, which led to the temporary suspension of the use of this vaccine while investigation of the vaccine was undertaken in several countries including Austria, Bulgaria, Cyprus, Denmark, France, Germany, The Netherlands, Norway, Iceland, Ireland, Estonia, Indonesia, Italy, Latvia, Lithuania, Luxembourg, Portugal, Slovenia, Spain, Sweden, and Thailand (Agencies, 2021; Wise, 2021).

There are 7.01 million confirmed COVID-19 death cases as of January 2024, and the mortality risk of COVID-19 infection should be taken into consideration when evaluating the significant and rare adverse events reported. Another consideration to note is the total population being treated (13.53 billion doses have been administered globally) and those who have been vaccinated without experiencing serious adverse events or any adverse events. At present, 70.6% of the world population (i.e., 5.71 billion people) in 218 countries has received at least one dose of the COVID-19 vaccine (Mathieu, et al., 2020).

The COVID-19 pandemic was an unprecedented time for drug manufacturers. Manufacturers of COVID-19 vaccines had multifaceted challenges to overcome, such as upscaling vaccine production to meet supply (and quickly while maintaining product quality), supply of raw materials in the midst of national lockdown, management of clinical trials, and resolving new remote ways of working and limited resources onsite. Regarding pharmacovigilance, MAHs and regulatory authorities were working closely and independently to assess available information and publish relevant information as soon as possible, as there was tremendous public interest and very high media coverage.

The national COVID-19 vaccination programmes and heightened awareness of safety concerns have led to a very high volume of adverse event reporting and significantly impacted the MAHs' pharmacovigilance system. One aspect in particular was safety case management due to the increased volume of adverse event reporting that would have resulted in a backlog of safety cases for processing while the MAH sought additional resources and adequately trained pharmacovigilance specialists. In addition to the high volume, many safety case reports would lack sufficient details, resulting in a high possibility of duplicate cases, which can impact signal surveillance activities (increased interference and noise).

All this is done while maintaining routine activities for other products in the organisation's product portfolio.

Valproate

Another instance of applying pharmacovigilance involves the restricted use of valproate during pregnancy or in any woman or girl of childbearing age, unless the conditions of a new pregnancy prevention programme are met. Valproate-containing medicines have been approved nationally in the EU and many other regions to treat epilepsy and bipolar disorder and for the prevention of migraine. It is one of the most widely prescribed antiepileptic drugs globally. However, it has been established that if taken during pregnancy, it can affect the unborn baby and cause abnormalities or birth defects (EMA, European Medicines Agency, 2017a, b).

Upon recognising this risk, regulatory authorities globally implemented measures to minimise the associated risk through different risk minimisation measures, as follows: On 21 March 2018, the Coordination Group for Mutual Recognition and Decentralised Procedures (CMDh), a regulatory body comprising national regulatory authorities from EU member states, introduced stringent measures. These measures include prohibiting the use of valproate and related medicines for treating migraine or bipolar disorder during pregnancy. Treating epilepsy during pregnancy is allowed only if two specialists independently determine and document that no other effective treatment exists. Other measures include adding a visual warning regarding the pregnancy risks on the packaging of the medicine and patient cards that are supplied to the patients (EMA, Valproate and Related Substances, 2018).

A month later, the MHRA also announced that valproate was banned for use by any woman or girl of childbearing age unless they were registered in a pregnancy prevention programme. The French Agency for the Safety of Medicines and Health Products (ANSM) acted by disseminating information about the risks associated with the use of valproate-containing medication in women and girls of childbearing potential and leading to an extensive information campaign (A. Degremont, 2018). Regulatory authorities in other regions, such as the U.S. FDA and the Australian Therapeutic Goods Administration (TGA), have also issued safety announcements cautioning against the use of valproate in women or girls of childbearing age. They emphasise reserving its use for non-seizure-related indications unless the drug is essential for the patient's medical condition on a case-by-case basis, accompanied by stronger warnings on the drug labels (FDA, 2013; TGA, 2018).

The rest of this chapter will focus on the key components of the pharmacovigilance system and its quality framework, as well as some key practical considerations.

Pharmacovigilance cannot succeed in a Silo

It is also important to recognise that a pharmacovigilance system often requires input and contributions from multidisciplinary teams, including those in legal, procurement, medical information, product quality, medical affairs, and clinical operations, to achieve the objectives of pharmacovigilance. Consequently, MAHs should establish a formalised framework, such as a Quality Management System (QMS), to ensure compliance with both regulatory standards and internal company requirements in the realm of pharmacovigilance.

Figure 10.1 *presents some of the key pharmacovigilance activities such as safety information collection, safety data processing and reporting, safety signal management and communication, periodic safety reporting, risk management activities and product labelling management, and lists some of the internal and external contributors and collaborators who may be required to participate. The list of stakeholders is not an extensive list, and the level of contributions from the multidisciplinary teams may vary between organisations, as well as the names and titles of the functions.*

Quality Management System (QMS) is the 'Superglue' to the Processes

A QMS is defined as a formalised system that documents processes, procedures, and responsibilities for achieving quality policies and objectives. A QMS helps coordinate and direct an organisation's activities to meet customer and regulatory requirements and improve its effectiveness and efficiency on a continuous basis (Quality, 2024). A well-established QMS is vital to engender confidence that the data is reliable and trustworthy, so it can meet legislative requirements and inform business decisions. Ultimately, it allows accurate information to be communicated to the public, patients,

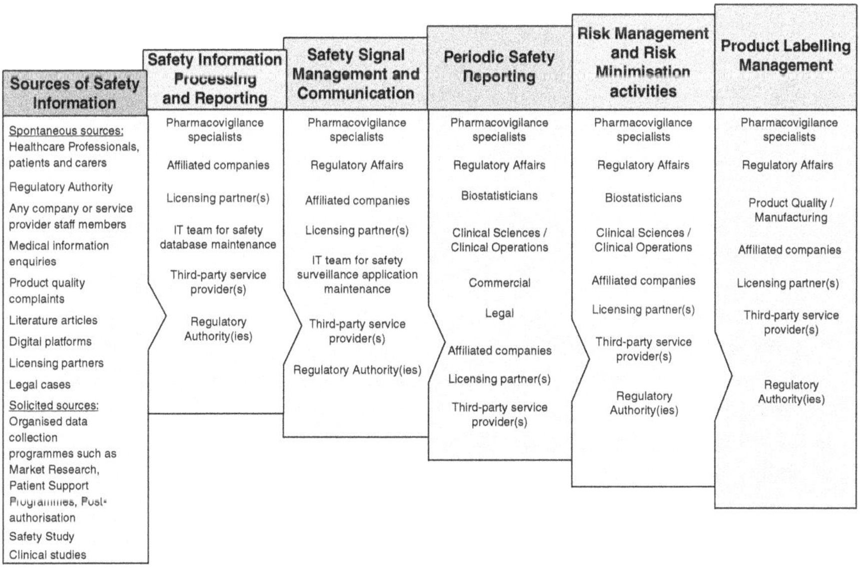

FIGURE 10.1 Examples of the multidisciplinary contributors and collaborators involved in the key pharmacovigilance activities.

and healthcare professionals (HCPs) to make informed decisions on taking a medical treatment.

Some of the key features of a pharmacovigilance QMS are described below:

- **Procedures Documents** – Instructions on how to carry out a GxP (regulated) activity, including identifying the responsible roles and expected timelines. Procedures may have a hierarchical structure and are commonly called Standard Operating Procedures (SOPs) and supported by Working Instructions or other more detailed step-by-step documents. This is to ensure the processes will be carried out consistently and as intended. Procedures should be regularly reviewed and updated as required.
- **Training and Qualification** – Established processes should be trained by relevant staff based on their job roles in a timely manner prior to performing the task. There may be additional considerations for qualification and training depending on the task to be performed, such as whether personnel are medically qualified to undertake a medical review of safety cases and their medical specialty.
- **Key Pharmacovigilance Personnel** – The Qualified Person for Pharmacovigilance (QPPV) is a mandatory position in some countries, and the QPPV is overall responsible for their organisation's pharmacovigilance system and has the autonomy to take appropriate actions to maintain an effective PV system. Their appointment may require registration or communication with the national regulatory authority. The QPPV qualification and availability requirements vary from country to country; for example, the appointed QPPV should be either a qualified physician or a pharmacist and available 24/7. Typically, the MAH may have a local safety officer or patient safety manager (titles may vary) responsible for a specific territory and be able to liaise with their regulatory authorities concerning pharmacovigilance activities and work closely with the QPPV.
- **Pharmacovigilance Training** – It is essential that all company (MAH) employees, including third-party service providers, receive general training in pharmacovigilance so all staff undertaking work for the MAH can recognise and report adverse events, including special situations such as pregnancy, lack of efficacy, occupational exposure, etc. This will ensure staff understand their responsibilities relating to safety information collection and reporting. The degree of training should be appropriate to the job role so that pharmacovigilance specialists involved in signal detection may undertake signal detection and signal management training, where appropriate.
- **Metrics and Compliance Monitoring** – Pharmacovigilance activities should be measured for compliance and have measurable key performance indicators defined for each activity. This will enable senior management to have an oversight of the performance of the pharmacovigilance system and allow senior managers to monitor for non-compliances and trends; this includes performance measurement of external pharmacovigilance licensing partners and service providers.

- **Change and Deviation Management** – Staff should be trained to recognise any deviations, changes, or non-compliance with any approved procedure or regulation. This will enable managing and correcting deviations in a timely manner according to internal procedures and, where necessary, implementing corrective actions and preventative actions (CAPAs) and effectiveness checks, as appropriate, to prevent reoccurrence. Management should have oversight of the level of compliance and deviations to ensure that the system is working as designed and meeting regulatory requirements.
- **Contract Management** – MAHs often have business collaborations with other MAHs, distribution partners for their products, and/or engage with service providers that may have aspects of pharmacovigilance activities such as case processing, literature monitoring, and conducting market research programmes. Therefore, the contractual terms between the parties should clearly outline each party's role and responsibilities relating to pharmacovigilance and regulatory activities.
- **Inspection Management** – Regulatory authorities may have inspection programmes to assess the compliance of a MAH's pharmacovigilance system with the country's regulations and licensing terms. There have been a growing number of regulatory authorities establishing a pharmacovigilance inspection programme.
- **Audit Management** – Audits are performed by the MAH to provide an independent assessment of their internal pharmacovigilance processes, relevant computerised systems, MAH-affiliated companies, and third parties such as service providers and licensing partners. Audits will evaluate the activities in scope against company procedures, contractual agreements, and regulations. Auditing is one way of providing oversight of the pharmacovigilance system to the MAH management team and the QPPV.
- **Record Retention** – Pharmacovigilance-related documents, whether in paper or electronic copy, should be retained as per the retention time required by the national requirements, e.g., MAHs should retain documentation for up to 15 years following the cessation of products marketed in the EEA. The MAH should ensure that there are appropriate security and physical measures in place to safeguard the documents that are in storage.
- **Business Continuity** – A backup plan should be established for protecting critical pharmacovigilance activities (as defined in GVP Module I), such as the continuous collection and reporting of safety information and the analysis and communication of safety signals. It should ensure minimal or no disruptions to the activity; the need for business continuity was highlighted by the COVID-19 pandemic situation and countries with unstable political situations.
- **Disaster Recovery** – The critical computerised systems used for pharmacovigilance-related activities should have regular backups of data (i.e., cloud storage and off-site computer servers) and escalation channels in place so that any system or power outage would be dealt with to ensure minimal disruption and restoration of key systems within an acceptable timeframe.

- **Key Pharmacovigilance System Description** – The Pharmacovigilance System Master File (PSMF) is a detailed description of the pharmacovigilance system of a MAH. It is usually a long document that presents an overview of the company's pharmacovigilance structure, processes, responsibilities, and key resources, including annexes covering sources of safety data, contractual agreements, CAPAs and deviations, pharmacovigilance system performance, etc. The content and format of the PSMF vary between countries, and some regulatory authorities may accept the EU PSMF with localised annexes. It is a key document to allow the QPPV to have oversight of the PV system as well as a commonly requested document by regulatory authorities as a prelude to a PV inspection. It is similar in principle to the site master file and the trial master file in GMP and GCP.

Key Pharmacovigilance Processes

Since MAHs are obligated to adhere to medicines legislation and adhere to applicable national pharmacovigilance regulations, they must consider many factors when designing and maintaining their pharmacovigilance system, such as the organisational set-up, size of the organisation, country(ies) of operation and regulatory landscape(s), the medicinal product (e.g., stage of development, drug class, therapeutic use, mechanism of action, formulary classification, etc.), intended treatment population (e.g., general population, special/high-risk populations, etc.), and whether they would use service providers for pharmacovigilance-related activities and the nature of the outsourced activities. There is no one size fits all, and MAHs must customise their pharmacovigilance system so key pharmacovigilance activities, as outlined below, can be designed and conducted according to their circumstances.

Safety Information Collection, Processing, and Reporting

Ensure safety information from all sources is collected and processed in a uniform and consistent manner (across all processing stages, e.g., data entry, coding of medical terms, medical assessments, and case narrative writing), and the safety information is reported to all relevant parties (e.g., contractual partners and regulatory authorities). The purpose of safety data collection is to enable the analysis of good-quality data, the timely identification of safety signals (i.e., risks) associated with the use of the medicinal product, and timely communication to various stakeholders. Communication with stakeholders could be performed *via* updating product labelling information and/or taking additional safety measures. Ultimately, healthcare professionals and patients should have all available information to make informed decisions about the use of the medicinal product.

Safety information can be received from various sources, either solicited (actively sought for by the MAH) or unsolicited (reported spontaneously). The channels set up for receiving safety information should ensure all potential incoming safety information (adverse events or other safety information) is reported to the pharmacovigilance department and processed accordingly without delay and in accordance with company procedures that meet regulatory requirements. Safety case reports may be referred to as Individual Case Safety Reports (ICSRs). It is crucial to identify and handle duplicate cases in the MAH's safety database to prevent overcounting of individual adverse drug reaction (ADR) reports and the exchange and reporting of repetitive information, which could lead to increased interference (noise) in signal detection performed by regulatory authorities and MAHs. Additionally, MAHs should ensure the processing of personal (sensitive) information recorded in safety case reports complies with the Data Protection Regulation in their respective territories, especially when sharing safety case information outside of the territory where the information originates or when the service provider involved is located outside of their jurisdiction.

Several factors could influence how safety information is handled and evaluated and whether additional measures should be in place. These factors may include:

- **Product Type and the Population being Treated** – For example, it is vital to follow up on the batch (lot) number of biological products to enable the identification of safety issues that may be related to a particular batch. Likewise, full traceability is needed for Advanced Therapy Medical Products (ATMPs) and other biological medicines such as gene therapy, somatic cell therapy, and tissue engineering products [i].
- **Indication of Medicinal Product** – For example, the timeline for reporting lack of effect cases associated with vaccines and contraceptive products to regulatory authorities would be shorter than the timeline for reporting lack of effect cases reported in association with generic medicinal products (in periodic safety reports).
- Medicinal products with risk(s) considered important, identified, important potential, and/or that are of special interest may have additional safety case processing requirements. For example, targeted safety (event) follow-up questionnaires could be used to gather structured information for a more informed consideration of the safety profile of the product.

Once safety case reports are processed, the MAH should submit ICSRs meeting the reporting criteria to applicable regulatory authorities within the timeframes stipulated. Additionally, the MAH will need to exchange safety information with their licensing partners as per the terms of the contractual agreement.

Safety Detection and Signal Management

Signal detection refers to the process of detecting any trends or safety signals that might indicate a previously unknown safety issue, including changes to what is known about the identified safety issue(s). The analysis should include all sources, such as ICSRs, literature publications, data from clinical and toxicology studies, and organised data collection programmes. The MAH should determine the appropriate methodological approach for their dataset; this may be using quantitative methods such as disproportionality scores and/or qualitative methods by reviewing pivotal individual case safety reports.

Potential signals should be taken through a formal process that includes validation, confirmation, analysis, prioritisation, assessment, and recommended actions. It is important for MAHs to maintain documentation of their signal detection and signal management activities. Key considerations in the methodology used will depend on the drug class, size of the dataset, treatment population, and stage of development, for example:

Marketing Status and Treatment Indication – For example, a newly launched medicinal product or those used in orphan indications may not have adequate case volume for a complex statistical methodology to be applied. In this situation, it might be more appropriate to use a qualitative approach. Vice versa, using only a qualitative approach might not be suitable for a well-established product or a product with a high volume of ICSRs.

Development Stage and Dataset Size – For example, the frequency of signal detection would be higher for a newly launched product or products with many clinical activities (e.g., weekly to biweekly) as opposed to established products with no ongoing clinical studies (e.g., biannually to annually).

Periodic Safety Reporting

Periodic safety reports provide a comprehensive overview of the safety profile of a medicinal product at predefined intervals, presenting cumulative and interim analyses for developmental and marketed medicinal products. The documents are required by many regulatory authorities to summarise the collected safety data, including new or emerging risks, and assess the benefit-risk balance.

The type of periodic safety report for investigational products in clinical development is known as a Development Safety Update Report (DSUR) and is known as a Periodic Benefit Risk Evaluation Report (PBRER) [ii] in the EU or a Periodic Adverse Drug Experience Report (PADER) in the U.S. for marketed products. The submission of periodic safety reports will follow the submission schedule set by the regulatory authorities or the conditions stipulated with the marketing approval, usually dependent on the safety profile of the product, its characteristics, and its stage in the product's life. There is a specific format for these reports, and often other regulatory authorities may agree to accept the EU format with a localised appendix and/or covering letter.

The authoring of a periodic safety report often requires input from other departments outside of pharmacovigilance, such as regulatory affairs, clinical development teams, commercial teams, and affiliated companies, as applicable.

Risk Management and Risk Minimisation Measures

Risk management activities are strategies that are implemented to reduce the risks associated with a medicinal product. In the EU, risk management activities are described in a comprehensive document named 'Risk Management Plan' (RMP), which is usually developed at the time of submission of the initial Marketing Authorization Application (MAA).

The RMP contains three main sections: (i) Safety Specification; (ii) Pharmacovigilance Plan; and (iii) Risk Minimisation Measures. The RMP starts with what is known to the MAH about the target population and epidemiology of the indication(s) of the product, clinical data (and populations not studied), post-authorisation experience, identified and potential risks, and a summary of safety concerns. This leads to an outline of the pharmacovigilance plan and risk minimisation measures for the product taken by the MAH. By doing so, this is a proactive approach to managing the risks associated with the product throughout its lifecycle, from pre-authorisation to post-authorisation stages. Examples of routine risk minimisation measures may be the legal status of the medicinal product, i.e., over-the-counter or prescription only; product labelling (such as the use of label warnings); and routine PV activities (such as periodic safety reporting). Additional risk minimisation measures (aRMMs) could include controlled access programs or educational programs where educational materials such as HCP brochures and patient leaflets are provided to healthcare professionals and patients, respectively; other aRMMs could be considered by the MAHs. Ultimately, the MAH should implement the appropriate risk minimisation measures to ensure the safe and effective use of their medicinal products.

Unlike the US, risk management planning is in the form of a Risk Evaluation and Mitigation Strategy (REMS) that may be required for some medicinal products (mainly prescription drugs and biologics but can include generic prescription medications), excluding over-the-counter medication. The purpose of the REMS is to address a specific known or potential serious safety concern with the medicinal product and support the US FDA decision to approve the product to remain on the market.

Another note is that the information on the potential and identified safety risks presented in the product's RMP should align with what is presented in other documents, such as the periodic safety reports.

Product Labelling

Medicinal product labelling (packaging and package leaflet/insert) contains information for the safe and effective use of the medicinal product and is based on a country's legal and regulatory requirements. Information to be presented in the labelling typically includes the name of the medicinal product, its strength and pharmaceutical form, a statement of the active substances, the pharmaceutical form and contents, dose, quantity, method of administration, batch number, expiry date, storage and disposal information, and the name and address of the manufacturer or representative. The EU requirements on labelling and package leaflets are outlined in Directive 2001/83EC.

When a new or a change in a known safety signal has been validated through the safety signal detection and signal management process, the product labelling should be updated in a timely manner so the information is available to HCPs and patients for informed decision-making about the use of the medicinal product. HCPs should only use medicines outside their authorised indications when there are no suitable alternatives, and they should inform patients about the potential risks and benefits of such use.

The timeline for labelling updates and implementation into product packaging should be appropriate to the level of the safety risk.

In the EU, the product labelling document is known as the Summary of Product Characteristics (SmPC), and in other parts of the world, the document is known by other names such as the Prescribing Information, Product Information, or Product Monograph. The respective regulatory authority will review and approve the product labelling document before authorising its implementation into a new batch of medicinal products.

The management of the latest labelling information into product packaging often requires input from other departments outside of pharmacovigilance, such as regulatory affairs and manufacturing.

Safety Communication

Safety communication is a broad term in the EU to cover all types of information on a medicine made available to the public. This may include the topics discussed above, such as the product labelling, routine, and additional risk minimisation material(s) produced and published by the MAHs or on a company's websites. Additionally, safety communication may also refer to the public assessment reports produced and published by regulatory authorities.

A summary of the key pharmacovigilance activities and the general workflow steps is shown in Figure 10.2.

Figure 10.2 presents some of the key pharmacovigilance activities, such as safety information collection, safety information processing and reporting, safety signal management and communication, periodic safety reporting, risk management activities, and product labeling management. For each pharmacovigilance activity, a list of general process steps and activities that may be utilised and incorporated into the activity workflow is shown to highlight the intricacies of each activity. The list of general process steps is not an extensive list, and the implementation of the steps and terms used may vary between organisations according to their situation.

Computerised Systems and Electronic Tools

Another important aspect is the use of electronic tools and computerised systems that have optimised pharmacovigilance activities and processes. It is an integral

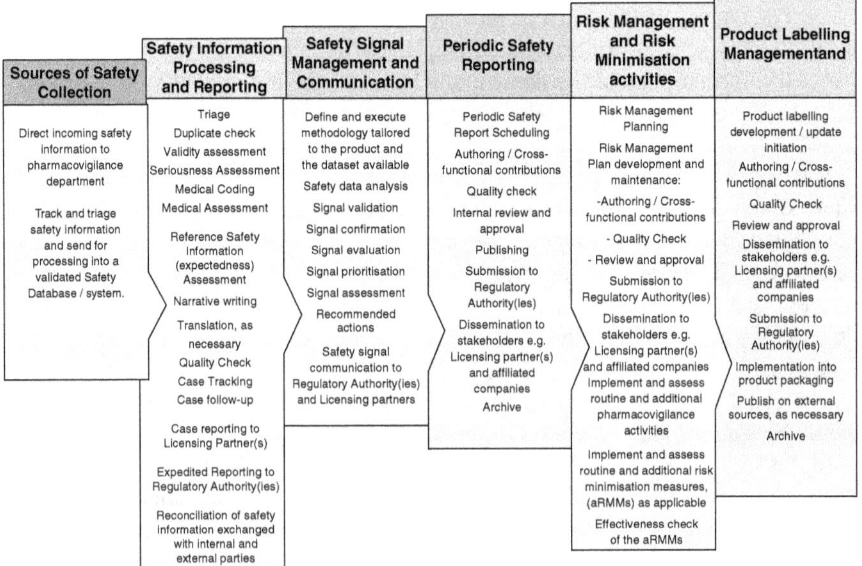

FIGURE 10.2 A simplified general workflow and process steps for key pharmacovigilance activities.

part of pharmacovigilance. Most, if not all, pharmacovigilance tasks are performed electronically, while some pharmacovigilance activities require complex and 'bespoke' electronic tools to enable the MAH to manage, manipulate, and retain large volumes of data.

Common computerised systems used for pharmacovigilance include a safety database for processing and submission of safety case reports and statistical software for data mining and interrogating the safety data. Therefore, it is essential to implement and maintain validated computerised systems for regulated GxP activities.

Another aspect is that the computerised systems are often multifaceted and able to "speak" to other computerised systems. For example, safety case reports received *via* the databases for medical information enquiry and product quality could be transferred to the safety database if the validated computerised systems are set up to do so. In addition, MAHs should ensure interactions with external third parties' systems to ensure accurate and timely case reporting and exchange *via* online portals or gateways with contractual partners and regulatory authorities.

One area where there have been tremendous advancements in pharmacovigilance is the use of artificial intelligence (AI) and machine learning (ML) to enable various computerised systems to be automated and work closely together. For instance, safety case management may include automation of the mapping of source documents into relevant fields in the safety database, medical coding of reported adverse events, auto-translation, and auto-population of safety case narratives. Besides this, technology has sped up the process of detecting adverse drug events and other drug-related issues by using predictive analytics, natural language processing (NLP) algorithms, and machine learning models. AI and ML can help detect potential adverse drug events that may have been overlooked by traditional methods. Additionally, AI and ML are being used to find patterns in drug use and potential drug interactions that could lead to potential safety issues and potential drug interactions, helping to reduce the risk of drug-related adverse events.

This relieves pharmacovigilance specialists from the administrative work, which can be error-prone and require effective quality check steps, which further adds to the administrative burden. Other benefits include faster processing times and improved consistency and quality. AI and ML can enable smarter ways of working by allowing PV specialists to focus on the more difficult cases, medical assessments, and other process improvement activities.

Final Thoughts...

Safety data collected in clinical studies is limited because of the size and composition of the participants, but it determines the safety profile, warnings, and usage limitations when marketed. As the product is launched, more critical data may indicate and warrant further label (product information) changes and notification to prescribers. As usage broadens through authorisations across the world, the safety profile can change due to various patient factors and an increase in the number of doses administered.

Pharmacovigilance plays a crucial role in ensuring the safety of medicinal products on the market through continuous monitoring of safety data to make timely updates to product information and communicate with stakeholders when appropriate. As such, the design and maintenance of the pharmacovigilance system may need to be reviewed and adjusted accordingly as the organisation changes over time to ensure its appropriateness and effectiveness. These efforts contribute to informed decision-making by both patients and prescribers, leading to improved patient care. This is particularly significant in scenarios where no alternative treatments exist or when significant risks can be managed so that the therapeutic benefits of a product outweigh its risks.

ACKNOWLEDGEMENTS

I am deeply thankful to my PV experts and dear friends, Morell David and Sylvia Kranich, both possessing extensive GxP expertise, for their invaluable feedback and shaping of this chapter. I also extend my appreciation to Gavin Hackett, whose input greatly contributed to refining this chapter.

NOTE

1 In the EU, the product labelling document is known as the Summary of Product Characteristics (SmPC), and in other parts of the world the document is known by other names such as the Prescribing Information, Product Information or Product Monograph. These documents can be updated with new safety and efficacy data from clinical trials, changes in undesirable effects, new warnings, drug-drug interactions, and information regarding shelf life and/or storage conditions.

BIBLIOGRAPHY

A. Degremont, B. L. (2018). Impact of the French Agency for the Safety of Medicines and Health Products communication on sodium valproate prescription in women of childbearing potential age. *Revue d'Épidémiologie et de Santé Publique*, *66*(5), S426–S427.

Agencies, A. J. (2021, March 15). *Which Countries have Stopped Using AstraZeneca's COVID Vaccine?* Retrieved May 01, 2023, from: https://www.aljazeera.com/news/2021/3/15/which-countries-have-halted-use-of-astrazenecas-covid-vaccine#:~:text=Sweden%20and%20Latvia%20on%20Tuesday,and%20The%20Netherlands%2C%20among%20others.

Ahmad, S. R. (2003). Adverse drug event monitoring at the Food and Drug Administration. *Journal of General Internal Medicine*, *18*(1), 57–60.

EMA. (2017). *European Commission Closes Infringement Procedure against Roche*. Retrieved May 01, 2023, from European Medicines Agency: https://www.ema.europa.eu/en/news/european-commission-closes-infringement-procedure-against-roche

EMA. (2017, September 26). *Public Hearing on Valproate: Summary of Safety Concerns and List of Questions for the Public Hearing*. Retrieved April 12, 2023, from European Medicines Agency: https://www.ema.europa.eu/en/documents/other/public-hearing-valproate-summary-safety-concerns-list-questions-public-hearing-valproate_en.pdf

EMA. (2018, June 07). *Valproate and Related Substances*. Retrieved April 12, 2023, from European Medicines Agency: https://www.ema.europa.eu/en/medicines/human/referrals/valproate-related-substances-0

EMA. (2020, November 13). *Pharmacovigilance Plan of the EU Regulatory Network for COVID-19 Vaccines*. Retrieved 04 12, 2023, from European Medicines Agency: https://www.ema.europa.eu/en/documents/other/pharmacovigilance-plan-eu-regulatory-network-covid-19-vaccines_en.pdf

EMA. (2022, March 14). *Introductory Cover Note, Last Updated with Release of Addendum III of Module XVI on Pregnancy Prevention Programmes for Public Consultation*. Retrieved March 14, 2023, from European Medicines Agency: https://www.ema.europa.eu/en/documents/regulatory-procedural-guideline/guidelines-good-pharmacovigilance-practices-gvp-introductory-cover-note-last-updated-release_en.pdf

EMA. (2023, April 11). *Pharmacovigilance: Overview*. Retrieved from European Medicines Agency: https://www.ema.europa.eu/en/human-regulatory/overview/pharmacovigilance-overview

FDA. (2013, May 06). *FDA Drug Safety Communication: Valproate Anti-Seizure Products Contraindicated for Migraine Prevention in Pregnant Women due to Decreased IQ Scores in Exposed Children*. Retrieved from US Food and Drug Administration: https://www.fda.gov/drugs/drug-safety-and-availability/fda-drug-safety-communication-valproate-anti-seizure-products-contraindicated-migraine-prevention

Giulia Fornasier, S. F. (2018). An historical overview over pharmacovigilance. *International Journal of Clinical Pharmacy*, *40*, 744–747.

ICH. (2023, October 25). *Mission: Harmonisation for Better Health*. Retrieved from The International Council for Harmonisation of Technical Requirements for Pharmaceuticals for Human Use (ICH): https://www.ich.org/page/mission

International Society of Pharmacovigilance. (2023, April 11). *ISoP*. Retrieved April 11, 2023, from: https://isoponline.org/about-isop/

Kim, J. H. & Scialli, A. R. (2011). Thalidomide: The tragedy of birth defects and the effective treatment of disease. *Toxicological Sciences: An Official Journal of the Society of Toxicology*, *122*(1), 1–6.

Loke, S. S. (2012). Drug safety assessment in clinical trials: Methodological challenges and opportunities. *Trials 13*, 138.

Mathieu, E., Ritchie, H., Rodés-Guirao, L., Appel, C., Giattino, C., Hasell, J., … Roser, M. (2020). *Our World in Data*. Retrieved from Coronavirus (COVID-19) Vaccinations: https://ourworldindata.org/covid-vaccinations

MHRA. (2020, December 21). *Guidance Note: Exceptions and Modifications to the EU Guidance on Good Pharmacovigilance Practices that Apply to UK Marketing Authorisation Holders and the Licensing Authority*. Retrieved May 01, 2023, from Medicines & Healthcare Products Regulatory Agency: https://www.gov.uk/government/publications/exceptions-and-modifications-to-the-eu-guidance-on-good-pharmacovigilance-practices-that-will-apply-to-uk-mahs-and-the-mhra

NBER. (2023, August). *FDA Adverse Event Reporting System*. Retrieved from National Bureau of Economic Research: https://www.nber.org/research/data/fda-adverse-event-reporting-system

Prevention, C. F. (2023). *Selected Adverse Events Reported after COVID-19 Vaccination*. Retrieved April 12, 2023, from https://www.cdc.gov/coronavirus/2019-ncov/vaccines/safety/adverse-events.html

Ronald Mann, E. B. (2007). *Pharmacovigilance*, 2nd Edition. Chichester: John Wiley & Sons, Ltd.

Sabine Jeck-Thole, B. E. (2023). *The Future of Pharmacovigilance: The Right Positioning of Pharmacovigilance is a Key Enabler in Drug Development*. Boston: Arthur D. Little.

Sonawane, K. B., Cheng, N., & Hansen, R. A. (2018). Serious adverse drug events reported to the FDA: Analysis of the FDA adverse event reporting system 2006-2014 database. *Journal of Managed Care & Specialty Pharmacy*, *24*(7), 682–690.

TGA. (2018, July 04). *Advisory Committee on Medicines (ACM) Meeting Statement, Meeting 9, 31 May–1 June 2018*. Retrieved from Therapeutic Goods Administration Australian Government: Department of Health and Aged Care: https://www.tga.gov.au/sites/default/files/acm-meeting-statement-meeting-9-31-may-1-june-2018.pdf

Uppsala Monitoring Centre. (2023, April 11). *UMC*. Retrieved from Uppsala Monitoring Centre: https://who-umc.org/about-the-who-programme-for-international-drug-monitoring/

Vargesson, N. (2015). Thalidomide-induced teratogenesis: History and mechanisms. *Birth Defects Research Part C: Embryo Today: Reviews*, *105*(2), 140–156.

Waqas, R., Arfons, L. M., & Lazarus, H. M. (2011). The rise, fall and subsequent triumph of thalidomide: Lessons learned in drug development. *Therapeutic Advances in Hematology*, *2*(5), 291–308.

WHO. (2023, March 13). *Global Convening on COVID-19 Vaccination Monitoring and Related System Strengthening*. Retrieved April 12, 2023, from World Health Organisation: https://www.who.int/news-room/events/detail/2023/03/13/default-calendar/global-convening-on-covid-19-vaccination-monitoring-and-related-system-strengthening

WHO. (2023, October 25). *Regulation and Prequalification*. Retrieved from World Health Organisation: https://www.who.int/teams/regulation-prequalification/regulation-and-safety/pharmacovigilance

Wise, J. (2021). Covid-19: European countries suspend use of Oxford-AstraZeneca vaccine after reports of blood clots. *British Medical Journal*, *372*, 699.

11 Electronic Records; Electronic Signature and Data Integrity

Randall Basinger

In 1997, when Paul Motise, an FDA investigator, and a team of colleagues at the US FDA were drafting what would become Part 11, the information technology landscape looked very different than it does today. With the regulation, they were navigating a world where open Excel files were used for data capture and transfer, and many systems utilized shared login and password combinations. And similarly, another 30 years out from today, the technology landscape for clinical trials is likely to look very different than it does today. That is one of the things that makes the last 27 years under 21 CFR Part 11 and its European counterpart, Annex 11: Computerised Systems, so amazing to reflect on. While there has been some updated guidance regarding the way that the regulation should be applied during the last 27 years, the core tenants of the regulation have withstood and evolved with the technology with which it is to be applied.

At one point in my career and early in the life of the regulation, I was asked by my boss to provide an assessment of what could be left out of the regulation for a "lite" approach to Part 11. After sitting down with my team and building out a risk and impact assessment of what would be "optional" with the removal of each requirement, I went back to see my boss with the answer.

"So what would you leave out in a lite approach?" she asked.

"Nothing," I replied. "We ran the assessment and there is nothing that we would take out of the requirements in the regulation in order to gain a 'lite' approach. Each of the requirements – access control, audit trails, validation of the system functionality – provides a unique control for data integrity. Remove even one requirement and you start impacting the data integrity from that system."

"Okay," she said, thanking me for providing the spreadsheet with each of the requirements and the associated risk encountered with the removal of each one.

As I got up to leave her office, I turned around. "There is one thing that we felt could be left out."

"Yeah. What is that?"

"The requirement for a certification letter submitted to the FDA detailing an organization's intent to utilize electronic signatures," I said. "If you neglected to send that into the agency, they could 'ding' (cite) you for not following the requirement in the regulation, but it would not necessarily impact the integrity of the data if you followed the other requirements for confirming the e-signature controls that are outlined there."

DOI: 10.1201/9781003407010-11

"Noted," she said, and let me leave her office before getting on the phone and informing those inquiring about a potential "lite" approach to Part 11 that they were putting the integrity of their data from the planned system at risk.

Interestingly enough, that certification letter is now the one thing that the FDA has updated since releasing the regulation in 1997. In 2023, they updated the address for where to send in the letter and also made the submission of a certification letter optional with the update. Other than that, the regulation and the expected controls detailed therein have maintained the same wording and expectations even as new technologies came along. The agency has updated the approach with various guidances (General Principles of Software Validation; Final Guidance for Industry and Staff, January 2002; Guidance for Industry Part 11, Electronic Records; Electronic Signatures – Scope and Application, August 2003; Policy for Device Software Functions and Mobile Medical Applications Guidance for Industry and Food and Drug Administration Staff, September 2022; and most recently, Computer Software Assurance for Production and Quality System Software, Draft Guidance, September 2022) on how to think about the latest tech tool used in clinical trials, with lab equipment, and in manufacturing systems.

Over the course of this chapter, the details of the regulatory requirements will be discussed, and the role that each plays in supporting data integrity will be addressed. Along the way, we will also touch on the iteration of the regulation with the upcoming Computer Software Assurance (or CSA) guidance (Computer Software Assurance for Production and Quality System Software, Draft Guidance, September 2022). That should emerge from the comment 'cocoon' that occurred in 2022 following its issuance for review and comment from the industry and explore a little where that may take the regulation as it moves deeper into its third decade of existence.

SUBPART B – ELECTRONIC RECORDS

At the heart of 21 CFR Part 11 is the following requirement:

11.10 (a) Validation of systems to ensure accuracy, reliability, consistent intended performance, and the ability to discern invalid or altered records.

Back in 1997, the internet had come on the scene with the introduction of broadband connections. Computers were starting to 'talk' to each other. The first electronic mail (email) systems were active, paving the way for electronic-based communication. While the term validation was in use in the pharmaceutical research, laboratory and manufacturing industry; and use of an Installation Qualification (IQ), Operational Qualification (OQ) and Performance Qualification (PQ) had been defined (section 3.3.3 and definitions, General Principles of Software Validation; Final Guidance for Industry and FDA Staff, January 2002) by the industry dating back to the initial predicate rules in the 1970s as a standard set of documentation and testing to support controlled and consistent performance of systems, the FDA was looking to codify the expectation that people test and demonstrate that the computer systems in use worked as they expected according to a defined set of requirements. Utilizing the processes that had been popping up in the industry, the agency would follow up on Part 11 with guidance (see earlier references to guidance provided) outlining the role of drafting requirements and performing documented testing and evidence to demonstrate that the system and functionality in question performed as expected by the defined requirement known as User Requirement Specifications. This provided for accurate data output that the FDA could then utilize and rely upon for their assessment and drug approval processes. The reliability and consistent intended performance components of the requirement would become the current Disaster Recovery and Business Continuity plans and associated testing that proved for recovery of the system and data utilizing backup and recovery processes from backup tapes (now via online or cloud-based storage, typically), and the system should have ways to be able to confirm if an entry or data calculation is valid and not altered since the initial calculation or capture. Where a change was made to the data or calculation, there was expected to be a way to view or capture that change, i.e., an audit change, including who and when it was performed.

21CFR11.10 (e) Use of secure, computer-generated, time-stamped audit trails to independently record the date and time of operator entries and actions that create, modify, or delete electronic records. Record changes shall not obscure previously recorded information. Such audit documentation shall be retained for a period at least as long as that required for the subject electronic records and shall be available for agency review and copying.

At the time of the drafting of 21 CFR Part 11, many of the systems would allow users to make changes without the ability to easily detect the changes. Whereas paper records in the regulated space included standard controls for documenting changes to the data – a process of lining out the change, updating the data and then initialing and dating the change. Thus, changes on paper could be easily detected and were commonly known as 'Good Documentation Practices' embedded in a standard operating procedure widely used by all regulated industries. But now, with the computer environment and word processing, edits or data changes were done electronically, with no easy way to detect when, where, and by whom a change was made. This posed a real problem for the agency when it came to submissions. There was a potential open process for changes that they would not be able to detect. So the writers of Part 11 looked to define the expectation that the computer collecting data would expand the functionality of the system with functionality whose sole purpose was to capture the data change, who made the change, and when it was made, and they noted that the system should require the user to put in a reason for the change. This was a revolutionary idea, as most of the systems on the market did not include these types of controls, and the processing capacity and bandwidth of most systems at the time prevented this from being included. The industry 'barked loudly' about this change and the costs that it would incur to bring the systems up to standard. The FDA heard those cries and provided guidance (Guidance for Industry Part 11, Electronic Records; Electronic Signatures – Scope and Application, August 2003) for better defining the scope and the agency's application of Part 11 that allowed for a hybrid approach where if the system did not include an audit trail with the required functional elements, they would allow the industry time to upgrade systems, where necessary, or implement procedural controls to support data integrity. While not optimal, this put the industry on notice that they would be accountable for making sure that new systems included the ability to capture data changes via a system-based audit trail that captured details for the initial entry of the data and subsequently captured changes to the data so that someone reviewing an audit trail history or report for a piece of data could trace the current data back to its origins with a date and time for each change. This also necessitated that there be an information technology (IT) process for making sure the time and date stamp were synced to the system and that these two important elements were consistently synched for the accuracy of the system data.

As you can see from these two examples, the basic requirement tenants of Part 11 ended up with an expansion of required controls that began to be incorporated into functional testing/validation of systems as they were designed with the regulated expected controls. The below chart provides a list of each of the requirements and many of the current expected tests to demonstrate evidence of these controls and, thus, data integrity.

21 CFR PART 11 REQUIREMENTS AND ASSOCIATED TESTING CONTROLS FOR CONSIDERATION

Requirement	Expanded Testing Controls
11.10 (a) Validation of systems to ensure accuracy, reliability, consistent intended performance, and the ability to discern invalid or altered records	1. Testing traced to functional requirements. 2. Business continuity and disaster recovery planning and testing for the system. 3. Testing that demonstrated altered or invalid records.
11.10 (b) The ability to generate accurate and complete copies of records in both human-readable and electronic form suitable for inspection, review, and copying by the agency.	1. Demonstrate the ability to print or copy accurate records from the system. 2. Records should contain the audit trail history for the data to be included and reviewed.
11.10 (c) Protection of records to enable their accurate and ready retrieval throughout the record retention period.	1. Demonstrate the ability to retrieve records to the extent of expected record retention. 2. Demonstration and testing of system backups and evidence of monitoring for backup alerts or failures. 3. Business continuity and disaster recovery planning and testing for the system for the protection of records.
11.10 (d) Limiting system access to authorized individuals.	1. Demonstration and testing of role-based access and controls (positive access and negative rejection of access). 2. System must force a change of password and require password changes at an established frequency. 3. Testing of functionality for password reset or forgotten password that prevents someone else from knowing the password. 4. System will automatically log someone out after a period of inactivity. 5. System will automatically disable a user's account after a specified period of non-use or a defined number of invalid attempts to access the system.

(Continued)

(Continued)

Requirement	Expanded Testing Controls
	6. User will not be able to log into the system with disabled account credentials. 7. System will provide the ability to activate and deactivate user accounts.
11.10 (e) Use of secure, computer-generated, time-stamped audit trails to independently record the date and time of operator entries and actions that create, modify, or delete electronic records. Record changes shall not obscure previously recorded information. Such audit trail documentation shall be retained for a period at least as long as that required for the subject electronic records and shall be available for agency review and copying.	1. Demonstration that the system time is synced to a standard time in the system and cannot be altered by the user. 2. Demonstration and testing to confirm that an audit trail is recorded for each record field required. 3. Demonstration and testing that the user cannot turn-off or turn on audit trails. 4. Audit trial must show the name of the person performing the entry or update, the data and time of the entry, and the reason for the change to the entry. 5. Demonstration that the audit trail can be printed or copied for an inspector to take with them. Generally, this can be a validated report that should be confirmed to be accurate and complete when validated.
11.10 (f) Use of operational system checks to enforce permitted sequencing of steps and events, as appropriate	1. Demonstration that the system syncs the time and date to a central source that cannot be changed by the general user.
11.10 (g) Use of authority checks to ensure that only authorized individuals can use the system, electronically sign a record, access the operation or computer system input or output device, alter a record, or perform the operation at hand.	1. Testing to demonstrate that the role-based access that has been set up for the system is correct for the given roles. 2. Testing that when a person doesn't have appropriate access to the system, the role cannot access the system. 3. System should be tested to demonstrate that there is a process for granting and revoking access and that the organization's processes demonstrate the appropriate authorization to grant access.
11.10 (h) Use of device (e.g., terminal) checks to determine, as appropriate, the validity of the source of data input or operational instruction.	1. Though most organizations no longer use devices like Secure ID cards/tokens, many are going to use two-factor authentication with mobile phones or controlled single sign-on services, and those processes and services should be tested to demonstrate appropriate access control.
11.10 (i) Determination that persons who develop, maintain, or use electronic record/electronic signature systems have the education, training, and experience to perform their assigned tasks.	1. Organizations should have documented training that confirms the users who are granted access have the appropriate training to support planned use of the functionality of the system. This can be challenging when you provide site users (principal investigators, sub-investigators, etc.) with system access and they need to have documented training on their planned use.

(Continued)

(Continued)

Requirement	Expanded Testing Controls
11.10 (j) The establishment of and adherence to written policies that hold individuals accountable and responsible for actions initiated under their electronic signatures in order to deter record and signature falsifications.	1. Companies should have procedures that outline their approach to the planned use of electronic signatures and a process of identity verification. Most companies utilize their HR processes for I9 employment as their verification, but this can be more of an issue when you are using sites that are not part of your organization during a clinical trial.
11.10 (k) Use of appropriate controls over system documentation, including: *(1) Adequate controls over the distribution of, access to, and use of documentation for system operation and maintenance.* *(2) Revision and change control procedures to maintain an audit trail that documents time-sequenced development and modification of system documentation.*	1. Use and leverage vendor documentation as well as an organization's own validation documentation for a system. In an inspection situation, organizations typically have an assigned system owner who manages the initial release and subsequent change control for the system, and all of the documentation must support evidence that the system works as intended during its operational use.
11.30 Controls for open systems. *Persons who use an open system to create, modify, maintain, or transmit electronic records shall employ procedures and controls designed to ensure the authenticity, integrity and, as appropriate, confidentiality of electronic records from the point of their creation to the point of their receipt. Such procedures and controls shall include those identified in 11.10, as appropriate, and additional measures such as document encryption and the use of appropriate digital signature standards to ensure, as necessary under the circumstances, record authenticity, integrity, and confidentiality.*	1. While many systems are now cloud-hosted with the hosting organizations being able to demonstrate controls and security via audits and reports, it is important that the internet-based transmission of data be demonstrated to have appropriate encryption for data privacy control for data in transit and at rest.
11.50 Signature Manifestations. *(a) Signed electronic records shall contain information associated with the signing that clearly indicates all of the following:* *(1) The printed name of the signer;* *(2) The date and time when the signature was executed; and* *(3) The meaning (such as review, approval, responsibility, or authorship) associated with the signature.*	1. Testing documentation should demonstrate that any signed records by the system include the printed name of the signer, the date and time of the signature execution, and the meaning (review, approval, responsibility, or authorship) of the document being signed. 2. All of the signature elements noted for a complete manifestation should be represented on the printed record as well as maintained on the printed record. 3. Testing that demonstrates that the signature is applied and retained with the signed record and cannot be excised, copied, or transferred elsewhere to be applied to other records.

(Continued)

(Continued)

Requirement	Expanded Testing Controls
(b) The items identified in paragraphs (a) (1), (a) (2), and (a) (3) of this section shall submit to the same controls as for electronic records and shall be included as part of any human-readable form of the electronic record (such as an electronic display or printout).	4. System testing or company procedures that make sure assigned user credentials (ID and password) are not reused or reassigned to someone else when an original assignee leaves the company. Accounts should be maintained as deactivated within the system as long as the system is in use.
11.70 Signature/record linking. *Electronic signatures and handwritten signatures executed on electronic records shall be linked to their respective electronic records to ensure that the signatures cannot be excised, copied, or otherwise transferred to falsify an electronic record by ordinary means.*	1. Testing should demonstrate that the signature applied to the record electronically remains only with that record and cannot be removed or copied/pasted to another record within the system.
11.100 General Requirements. *(a) Each electronic signature shall be unique to one individual and shall not be reused by, or reassigned to, anyone else.* *(b) Before an organization establishes, assigns, certifies, or otherwise sanctions an individual's electronic signature, or any element of such electronic signature, the organization shall verify the identity of the individual.* *(c) Persons using electronic signatures shall, prior to or at the time of such use, certify to the agency that the electronic signatures in their system, used on or after August 20, 1997, are intended to be the legally binding equivalent of traditional handwritten signatures.* *(1) The certification shall be signed with a traditional handwritten signature and submitted in electronic or paper form. Information on where to submit the certification can be found on the FDA's web page on Letters of Non-Repudiation Agreement.* *(2) Persons using electronic signatures shall, upon agency request, provide additional certification or testimony that a specific electronic signature is the legally binding equivalent of the signer's handwritten signature.*	1. Again, there should be a company process for access granting authorization, and the credentials should only be assigned to one person within the organization. 2. If a user leaves the organization, the account should be deactivated and the credentials should not be re-assigned to someone else. 3. Demonstration that, when a user returns, they are given the same reactivated credentials. 4. Testing that demonstrates for any period of continuous signing that the user utilizes both ID and password credentials on the first signing and only has to use the password on subsequent signings. Many organizations require the entry of both for any signing. 5. There was an initial requirement for a certification letter to the agency for the intended use of electronic signatures. This represented that there would be training for an organization's users on the importance of maintaining their electronic identity credentials. In 2023, the certification letter was made optional by the FDA, and they updated the submission address to: Jessica Bernhardt, Electronic Submissions Gateway, U.S. Food and Drug Administration, 3WFN, Rm. 7C34, 12225 Wilkins Ave., Rockville, MD 20852.

(Continued)

(Continued)

Requirement	Expanded Testing Controls
11.200 Electronic signature components and controls. *(a) Electronic signatures that are not based upon biometrics shall:* *(1) Employ at least two distinct identification components such as an identification code and password.* *(i) When an individual executes a series of signings during a single, continuous period of controlled system access, the first signing shall be executed using all electronic signature components; subsequent signings shall be executed using at least one electronic signature component that is only executable by, and designed to be used only by, the individual.* *(ii) When an individual executes one or more signings not performed during a single, continuous period of controlled system access, each signing shall be executed using all of the electronic signature components.* *(2) Be used only by their genuine owners; and* *(3) Be administered and executed to ensure that attempted use of an individual's electronic signature by anyone other than its genuine owner requires the collaboration of two or more individuals.* *(b) Electronic signatures based on biometrics shall be designed to ensure that they cannot be used by anyone other than their genuine owners.*	1. Demonstration by testing that electronic signatures are applied within the system with the use of two unique identifiers (user ID and password). 2. Demonstration that if a user returns, they are given the same reactivated credentials. 3. Testing that demonstrates for any period of continuous signing that the user utilizes both ID and password credentials on the first signing and only has to use the password on subsequent signings. Many organizations require the entry of both for any signing. 4. Organizations should have a process for periodic review of the access granted. In a recent EU guidance (Guideline on Computerised systems and Electronic Data in Clinical Trials, issued 09 Mar 2023/effective 09 Sep 2023) that went into effect in September 2023, the expectation of the review should also include those with elevated privileges (generally administrators), and the review of access logs and audit trail activities by those with elevated privileges should be reviewed to confirm that they are correctly using the activities and have not made unauthorized changes to data with their access, which can be harder to detect. 5. Any biometric access processes should be tested and validated with the system to demonstrate that they work as expected.
11.300 Controls for identification codes/ passwords. *Persons who use electronic signatures based on the use of identification codes in combination with passwords shall employ controls to ensure their security and integrity. Such controls shall include:* *(a) Maintaining the uniqueness of each combined identification code and password, such that no two individuals have the same combination of identification code and password*	1. Demonstration by testing that electronic signatures are applied within the system with the use of two unique identifiers (user ID and password). 2. Again, the expectation is that accounts be deactivated and not re-assigned to another user. 4. Demonstration that if a user returns, they are given the same reactivated credentials. 5. Management and validation of any tokens (such as Secure ID) or services (Okta) that provide additional credentials beyond the ID and password to grant access to the system.

(Continued)

(Continued)

Requirement	Expanded Testing Controls
(b) Ensuring that identification codes and password issuances are periodically checked, recalled or revised (e.g., to cover such events as password aging)	
(c) Following loss management procedures to electronically deauthorize lost, stolen, missing, or otherwise potentially compromised tokens, cards, and other devices that bear or generate identification code or password information and to issue temporary or permanent replacements using suitable, rigorous controls.	
(d) Use of transaction safeguards to prevent unauthorized use of passwords and/or identification codes, and to detect and report in an immediate and urgent manner any attempts at their unauthorized use of the system security unit, and, as appropriate, to organizational management.	
(e) Initial and periodic testing of devices, such as tokens or cards, that bear or generate identification code or password information to ensure that they function properly and have not been altered in an unauthorized manner.	

Failure to appropriately validate and demonstrate that these expected system controls exist for systems involved with the submission of data to the FDA has resulted in warning letters for industry over the years, many focused on manufacturing and laboratory instruments. Some examples include the following:

1. Warning Letter September 26, 2023 noted the following: "In your written response, you acknowledged that Subject **(b)(6)** did not have e-Diary entries for **(b)(4)** to support eligibility. You indicated that as part of your corrective and preventive action plan, you will update your periodic review process to verify that subject e-Diary entries include the information required by the protocol."
2. Warning Letter August 17, 2023 noted the following: "You failed to verify or validate the ZYTO Hand Cradle GSR and associated proprietary software…Your Quality Supervisor stated your firm has no documented evidence to provide to demonstrate this testing was actually performed. She further stated you have no evidence to verify that design outputs meet design inputs…(and) Your firm's attorney stated that you have no documented validation of virtual items in the ZYTO software. Your firm also received a complaint of an "abnormal" or "empty" scan…"

3. Warning Letter December 02, 2022 noted the following: "you did not provide a CAPA plan with interim controls to prevent data and file deletion or modification until your **(b)(4)** is updated or how you will manage instruments that cannot transfer data."
4. Warning Letter to December 08, 2022 noted the following: "**Failure to exercise sufficient controls over computerized systems to prevent unauthorized access or changes to data, and failure to have adequate controls to prevent omission of data.** Your firm did not have system security and access control over its electronic data and software systems. Your analysts had access to delete and overwrite data. Our investigator observed over 100 deleted files in the recycle bins on the infrared (IR) spectrophotometer computer and on the ultraviolet-visible (UV-Vis) spectrophotometer computer. Specifically, multiple deleted analytical files had batch numbers in the filename and included files related to **(b)(4)** API, which your firm exports to the United States. The investigator also observed that the stand-alone computer systems for your UV-Vis and IR spectrophotometers failed to have usernames attributable to specific individuals and instead used a common username. No password was required to sign into the Windows operating system, nor did the analytical software require any additional user to log in. Furthermore, you did not back up your stand-alone computers used to operate your UV-Vis and IR spectrophotometers. To ensure data integrity, actions performed must be attributable to a specific individual in your CGMP computer systems, and equipment should be appropriately controlled to prevent deletion and/or changes except by authorized personnel."

It is clear from these examples and the actual warning letters issued by the US FDA that the lack of computer system validation and/or the demonstration of the appropriate system controls noted in the requirement table earlier in this chapter can lead the agency to question the integrity of data from a system.

And as the technologies continue to evolve, persons involved with the validation of computer systems for use in clinical trials should keep up with guidance and warning letters that are issued to address new software and systems that are introduced for use and do their best to align practices and system functionality to the requirements.

One area that has become important for organizations to demonstrate data integrity is audit trail review. Following the expectation for 15 or so years that systems implement appropriate audit trails for the systems used in clinical investigations, both the US FDA and EU EMA and MHRA began presenting an expectation that audit trails be reviewed at some periodic timing. Much like the original regulations, the industry has taken some time to discuss and digest these requirements, and you are seeing organizations develop processes for audit trail reviews (including activities like data management query reviews and source data reviews by monitoring staff). These reviews are intended to look for any anomalous data that may be identified through the review and incidents logged to get those anomalies addressed and corrected to maintain data integrity. Many organizations have now begun using machine learning algorithms to train software programs to look for these anomalies and aid in the targeting of data integrity concerns. It is expected that more of this will occur as we move into the future.

THE FUTURE – COMPUTER SOFTWARE ASSURANCE (CSA)

For years, the pharmaceutical industry has complained about the amount of documentation, validation testing, and the capture of screen shots as evidence, touting the fact that in recent years there have been testing systems and processes that provide for a more robustly controlled release process that leverages the tools and, in many cases, automated testing. As a result, in 2022, the US FDA issued a guidance (Computer Software Assurance for Production and Quality System Software, Draft Guidance, September 2022) outlining an approach to system validation that has become known as Computer Software Assurance or CSA. Within this guidance, which came out for comment and is back with the agency for updates based on the feedback from industry, they acknowledged that software processes had evolved to support good software practices and that risk assessments should also evolve and be utilized to demonstrate that risky functionality such as complex calculations, key functionality, or areas of systems that provide for important data needed for a submission or review should receive more attention in the development and validation testing than less risky components or functionality. So the risk assessment should then focus on the requirements of the system or change and the impact of those requirements captured in the risk assessment process.

The big challenge as the industry looks to adopt these processes is developing a risk assessment model that aids in the effective identification of risky or key areas of the system. While the ISO 14971 (International Standards Organization (ISO) 14971 Medical Devices – Application of Risk Management to Medical Devices) used largely within the medical device industry has provided for a well-worn risk assessment model as it supports the identification of harms associated with medical devices, the development of software and the importance of data integrity in clinical trial submissions ask for the model and considerations to be tailored to that effect. As the CSA model moves forward, it is going to be important to develop a risk assessment format and model that supports this and can be demonstrated throughout the CSA approach. For example, companies are starting to develop risk identifiers that are part of their traceability model so that the risks recognized in association with each requirement can start to build out a "risk heat map" for the software that supports where to apply challenge or more robust testing to make sure that bugs don't introduce risk to data integrity. The traceability matrix could look something like this for a test run:

Diagram 1:

Requirement	Risk Identifier	Test Case	Outcome	Comment
Requirement 1	RI1: High risk	Test Case 1 Test Case 2	Pass Fail	Fix, retested, and passed
Requirement 2	RI2: Medium risk	Test Case 1 or standard regression	Pass	
Requirement 3	RI3: Low risk	Regression testing only (or no testing)	Pass	

So again, the higher-risk areas of the software would get more or more focused testing, and by tagging it with a higher risk, developers and testers would know to pay more attention to Requirement 1 than Requirement 3. Software development tools and models have structured much of the software development these days to the point where software supporting these efforts can aid in the development of reports and metrics that provide ample evidence for demonstrating that software is being programmed and tested with quality in mind, with the goal of releasing software without defects or bugs as much as possible. Additionally, in the last few years, the speed of transmission and the internet/cloud-based connectedness of the software have allowed bugs to generally be quickly detected and addressed with an updated software release. All of these innovations have supported the regulator's belief that good software development practices can be reviewed and demonstrated to provide better confidence in the software used in clinical research. Thus, an integrated risk assessment model and demonstration of good testing and regression testing practices focused on identified risks are allowing for a better scaled testing model with details on testing execution available in summaries from manual and automated testing software, providing confidence in the quality of the software released. The key to success in CSA is the ability of the industry to develop an integrated risk assessment model that provides the information needed to make a risk-based decision that supports the release of quality software, and there is hope in the CSA guidance that this will result in more scalable testing and software development practices that are focused on the identified risks during the development or assessment of the planned change to any software.

12 Preparing for FDA Inspections at the Sponsor

Sandra "Sam" Sather, Tommy Lee, and Jennifer Lawyer

INTRODUCTION

From the discovery of the investigational product (IP) to pivotal trials, sponsors can invest hundreds of millions of dollars and years of personnel hours in the potential success of a New Drug Application (NDA). Recent data released from several studies suggest the total costs for the development of a new drug to approval have now surpassed an average of $2 billion US dollars, with a total of 55 NDA approvals in 2023. The NDA includes the entire story of the development of the drug from animal studies through pivotal trials, including study endpoint and safety data, information about the drug, packaging, and labeling, how the drug behaves in the human body, and information about reportable issues along the way. An NDA application triggers the Food and Drug Administration (FDA) into action to not only review the NDA application but also to investigate the sponsor and the entire program. The Agency will want to have a full understanding of the critical to quality processes that are in place, the sponsor's oversight of the clinical trial, and compliance with any other regulatory responsibilities. Every aspect of the NDA application is in scope for verification cross-functionally within the sponsor. This is accomplished through the Bioresearch Monitoring (BIMO) program, which monitors FDA-regulated clinical research through audits, inspections, and remote assessments.[1] After receipt of the marketing application, FDA field investigators are assigned to inspect the sponsor's clinical research sites, the sponsor and its oversight of services contracted out, and potentially the sponsor's vendors. Inspections can also occur for cause if an issue is suspected or reported.

BIMO COMPLIANCE PROGRAM GUIDANCE MANUALS (CPGM)

Each of the 11 BIMO Compliance Programs has guidance manuals (CPGM) that guide the FDA field investigators on how to conduct the inspection. The focus of this chapter is on Compliance Program Manual 7348.810 Sponsors and Contract Research Organizations.[2] The BIMO CPGMs are made publicly available because of the Freedom of Information Act of 1967, which improves transparency of government

DOI: 10.1201/9781003407010-12

activities by permitting public requests for documents, followed by the amendment in 1996, which allows documents to be delivered electronically, and the amendment in 2016, which allows appeals for denied requests.[3–5] BIMO CPGMs are regularly updated to address regulatory changes or changes in the agency's focus. For example, in 2021, the Sponsor/CRO CPGM included a whole new section for Outsourced Services and expanded sections relating to electronic systems, and likewise, inspections have an increased focus on sponsor oversight of their CROs and vendors. The FDA field investigator uses the BIMO CPGM as a playbook for document requests, process review, and interviewing the sponsor personnel.

HIGH PRIORITY TOPICS

Reviewing the BIMO CPGM line-by-line for inspection readiness would be a cumbersome task. Instead, a risk-based approach is warranted. High-priority topics are those that are Critical to Quality and impact the integrity of the clinical trial. According to ICH E8(R1) General Considerations for Clinical studies, Critical to Quality factors are those that support the safety and protection of participants, the reliability and quality of the study data, and the decisions made based upon the study results.[6]

Depending on the specifics of the program and the organization, sponsor functional areas should determine which BIMO CPGM topics are high priorities for their focused inspection readiness activities. Based upon the BIMO CPGM for Sponsors and CROs, the following are the main categories for determining the high-priority topics.

Outsourced Services/Vendor Oversight

Given the complexity of modern clinical trials and the systems required for trial oversight and conduct, sponsors regularly outsource activities to contract service providers (CSP), such as contract research organizations (CROs) and electronic systems vendors. When sponsors delegate responsibilities, the sponsor is responsible for oversight to ensure the CSP's compliance with regulatory requirements, adherence with Good Clinical Practice, and assurance that they are providing quality services and deliverables according to their delegated responsibilities.[2,7] The FDA field investigator would investigate the Sponsor's process for the contract service providers' selection and qualification/requalification, oversight of activities throughout the conduct of the trial, qualification and training of the CSP's personnel, communication, escalation, and management of issues, and the documentation of these oversight activities.

Clinical Investigator

Sponsors are responsible for ensuring the compliance of the clinical site with their regulatory responsibilities and their compliance with their processes and protocol. The focus of the sponsor BIMO inspection is on investigator and site selection, qualification and training of site personnel, oversight of investigator compliance, how any noncompliance was managed, and communication with clinical sites including providing safety updates.

Monitor Selection and Procedures

Oversight of the selection, training, and quality output of monitors is another high priority topic. Challenges include if there is a high turnover of monitors, monitors that were not qualified based upon experience and training, monitors that were terminated, or if the monitoring plan was not appropriately followed.

Safety Oversight

The sponsor should be able to demonstrate appropriate safety oversight including medical monitor oversight and a review of safety data for trends and reportable events. The sponsor would be asked who was responsible for implementing oversight and determining compliance with the applicable processes and plans. Sponsors/SME should be able to summarize the processes and procedures for the acquisition, handling, and review of safety data and the development of safety reports.

Safety and Adverse Event Reporting

The Agency would review when the sponsor became aware of Serious Adverse Events (SAEs) and if they were managed appropriately, including following reporting requirements to the Agency and ethics committees/IRBs. If SAEs go unreported or if there is a delay in reporting, the FDA could have a cause for concern for participant safety.

Electronic Records and Electronic Signatures

The Agency would investigate if electronic systems were in compliance with 21 CFR Part 11; systems were appropriately validated and kept in a validated state, had access control and audit trails, had processes in place to ensure data integrity and record retention, and so on. When electronic signatures are used, they need to be Part 11 compliant to verify they are unique to the user and the same as their wet ink signature. Review of FDA's Part 11, Electronic Records; Electronic Signatures – Scope and Application Guidance from September 2003 and Electronic Systems, Electronic Records, and Electronic Signatures in Clinical Investigations: Questions and Answers draft guidance from March 2023 can be beneficial to preparation activities.[8,9]

Data Collection and Handling

The FDA field investigator would be interested in the processes around the collection, management, analysis, and storage of study data, especially those that support primary or secondary endpoints or safety data that support the NDA. This topic frequently involves electronic systems such as Electronic Case Report Forms (eCRF),

Electronic Data Capture (EDC), Electronic Clinical Outcome Assessments (eCOA), and Electronic Patient Reported Outcomes (ePRO) and crosses into the high-priority topic above.

Investigational Product

The focus of an inspection at the sponsor would include sponsor processes and procedures to maintain IP integrity and manage end-to-end IP accountability. IP accountability is frequently maintained electronically by interactive response technology (IRT). If the sponsor utilizes a contract manufacturing organization (CMO) for manufacturing, packaging, labeling, and/or distribution, the agency would also be interested in the sponsor's oversight of contracted tasks.

Data and Safety Monitoring Board (DSMB)/ Data Monitoring Committee (DMC)

These external boards/committees often help in blinded trials and review study data for trends. If the sponsor chooses to have a DSMB or DMC, the FDA field investigator would request documentation of written operating procedures, the selection process of the members of the board/committee, and documentation of appropriate qualification and training of the members. The process that governs these activities is commonly documented in a charter that defines the specific requirements of the group. The SME for this topic should also know and be able to explain if and when unblinded data is reviewed.

Establishment Inspection Reports

If the sponsor has had previous regulatory inspections, reviewing the previously noted observations should take priority for inspection readiness activities. If the Agency notes that there was a previous concern that has not been adequately addressed or has recurred, it would be highly concerning. Sponsors should be able to describe what is being done differently, often captured in the form of a Corrective and Preventive Action (CAPA) plan, to ensure the issue does not reoccur. The CAPA plan should conduct a thorough diagnosis of the issues with root cause analysis and adequately address them through process changes that undergo planned effectiveness checks.

STORYBOARDING

After reviewing the high-priority topics from the sponsor BIMO CPGM, the functional areas should meet to review and discuss which are applicable to how the program was managed. The subject matter expert (SME) for the topic is identified and guides the creation of any inspection readiness tools they need to prepare to speak to the Agency. Storyboards are inspection readiness tools for the sponsor to document the history of the topic, who was involved during the course of the program or trial, which processes govern that topic (e.g. SOP, study specific plan, etc.), links to documentation, and times the process was not followed, when it was identified, and what was done. It is important to capture changes in processes or gaps that occurred during the timeframe. If a corrective and preventive action was needed, capture what remedial actions are being taken, who is overseeing the remedial actions, what changes have been made, if applicable, to ensure the issue does not arise again, and did it reoccur. Flow charts, timelines, or other visuals are helpful for an at-a-glance view of the process over time. Storyboards are used internally, or, in other words, are not shown to the Agency. Instead, they are preparation tools so that team members can have a better understanding of the process that occurred at the sponsor. This is especially helpful for transitions in personnel or in the case of the absence of the SME during an inspection. No one person should hold all the knowledge of this high-priority topic. Storyboards are also collaborative. When topics cross functional areas, storyboards can serve as instructional tools for the other functional areas. Sometimes inspection readiness tools are approved for use in an inspection. These are more commonly visual aids like flow charts, and organizational SOPs are provided to the Agency routinely. The Quality team needs to work closely with the functional area to ensure any tool that will be used by the Agency is appropriate and has been reviewed and approved for this use.

COACHING AND PRACTICE FOR BIMO INSPECTIONS

Once the high-priority topics have been chosen and storyboarded, SMEs for the appropriate topics should begin planning and practicing what they will say once the Agency arrives. The SMEs should be able to clearly and effectively explain their responsibilities, the steps and history of the process in question, what governs the process, and which documentation is available. Coaching on how to answer questions in a regulatory inspection should occur. Where applicable, personnel should know what electronic systems are used for their process and if they are compliant with 21 CFR Part 11, such as what measures are taken to ensure that the data is safeguarded against breaches or unauthorized access. It is important to be aware of gaps in critical processes and have a strategy in place for answering to the gaps. This can be strategized and practiced in advance.

During the interview, it is important to be calm, kind, and professional when interacting with a field investigator. It may reflect negatively if the response is panicked, angry, or defensive; be mindful of tone and facial expressions while answering questions. The field investigators are looking for an understanding of the sponsor's processes to get a better picture of what actually occurred. The SME should carefully listen to the questions and answer honestly to the best of their ability without any use of slang, excessive humor, or unnecessary elaborations. If the SME does not understand the question, they can ask for clarification, or they can rephrase the question back to the field investigator to get clarity. If the answer is unknown, or if the answer is a simple yes or no, then that should be the extent of their answer. If the topic moves into someone else's area of expertise, kindly defer to another SME. During the inspection, the ability to retrieve requested information, provide clarity to questions that arise within a reasonable amount of time, and leverage the end-of-day meetings with the auditor can be an opportunity to get an understanding of any open items to address for the next day of the inspection and potentially avoid an observation.

Practicing this during a mock is important to provide an opportunity to improve the hosting plan and backroom management.

Mock inspections are another useful tool for preparing for an inspection. By having someone play the part of the field investigator and using the BIMO CPGMs as a guide for the focus, the SMEs can have some practical experience in answering the questions. The mock investigator provides feedback on the sponsor's performance. Mock inspections should not be treated as a pass/fail endeavor but rather as a way to identify gaps, reflect on lessons learned, and plan next steps for improvements before the actual inspection.

DIFFERENT OUTCOMES OF A BIMO INSPECTION AND FDA 483 INSPECTIONAL OBSERVATIONS

Once the FDA field investigator has completed their inspection of the site, the data collected is reviewed and any observations noted, and within a few days they will share the results. If there were significant deviations from FDA regulations known as objectionable conditions, a FDA Form 483 is issued to the sponsor's senior management. The FDA Form 483 is not considered a final determination if the observations constitute violations of FDA regulations. This is discussed further in the 'Responses' section of this chapter.

The inspection results in one of three outcomes; no action indicated, voluntary action indicated, or official action indicated. No action indicated (NAI) means there were no objectionable practices or conditions observed; therefore no regulatory actions are needed and no 483 forms are issued. NAIs are the most common results in BIMO inspections (see Figure 12.1). Voluntary action indicated (VAI) means that

Sponsor/CRO Inspections
Final Classified FY 2017 – 2022

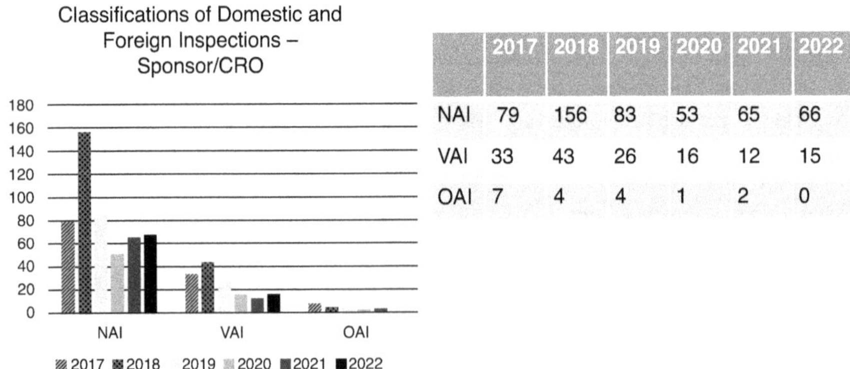

	2017	2018	2019	2020	2021	2022
NAI	79	156	83	53	65	66
VAI	33	43	26	16	12	15
OAI	7	4	4	1	2	0

FIGURE 12.1 BIMO sponsor/CRO inspection classifications from 2017 to 2022.

Source: FDA. *Bioresearch Monitoring (BIMO) Fiscal Year 2022 Metrics. Food and Drug Administration*. Retrieved 6 Feb 2024. URL: https://www.fda.gov/media/165853/download.

there were some objectionable practices and conditions that the sponsor should take actions to remediate; however, it does not require any regulatory actions to be taken by the Agency. Official action indicated (OAI) means that serious objectionable practices or conditions were observed that require remedial action but may also require FDA regulatory action or administrative sanctions. OAIs are relatively rare compared to NAI and VAI. For a history of reported 483s and the referenced regulations that were not followed, visit the FDA website for a list of inspectional observations dating back to 2006.[8]

For fiscal year 2022, BIMO observational trends show the top two sponsor observations were inadequate case histories and inadequate monitoring (see Figure 12.2).

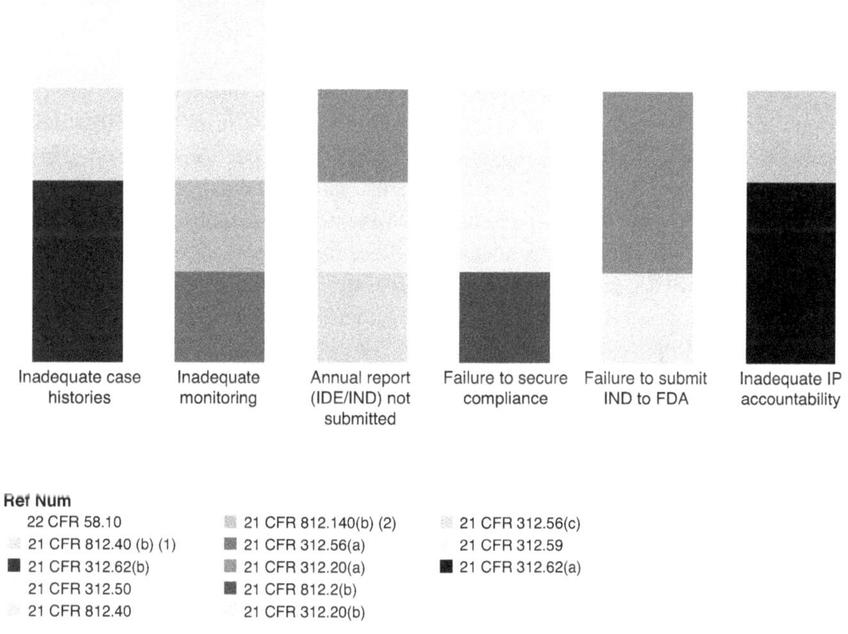

FIGURE 12.2 BIMO observational trends in sponsors in 2022.

Source: FDA. *FY 2022 Sponsor FDA 483 Observation Trends. Food and Drug Administration.* Retrieved 6 Feb 2024. URL: https://www.fda.gov/media/172781/download?attachment.

Responses

If the sponsor receives an FDA Form 483, they should take time to review and ensure the observations are fully understood. Ideally clarifications would have been requested during the inspection at the end of each day and at the closing meeting. Checking in with the inspector periodically during the audit and at the end of each day can provide an opportunity to assess what items they may plan to review, any areas where additional information may be required and time to further prepare. Sometimes the language in 483s does not contain enough information to identify the gap, so additional investigation may be warranted. Then the sponsor should investigate the root cause of the observations and determine the appropriate corrective and preventive action (CAPA) plan to implement. This includes immediate and long-term actions to prevent recurrence. Responses to observations should focus on the facts with evidence documented, the root cause of the deficiency, and what CAPAs will be in place to address the observations. A well written CAPA plan assures the Agency that the sponsor is taking the observations seriously and has a solid plan in place to address the Agency's concerns. Denial of observations is not warranted; however, if there was a misunderstanding, documentation of evidence that it was a misunderstanding can be provided with the response. Each observation should receive a response. Initial written responses are required within 15 days. If the FDA receives an adequate response to the FDA Form 483 within 15 business days after the inspection, it may positively impact the FDA's decision on further action needed. On the other hand, not responding may negatively impact the FDA's decision and reflect poorly on the sponsor.

Sponsors should also request the FDA Establishment Inspection Report (EIR), which is provided 3–6 months after the inspection; however, inspections that result in regulatory action would not be released until after the inspection is closed. The EIR is a detailed report of what the FDA field investigator did during the inspection, the sponsor's history, what was inspected, who was interviewed, observations that were made, and responses. The EIR is released to the sponsor's top management. Together, Form 483 and the EIR are the documentation of the evidence collected at the sponsor and any responses received. Periodic follow-up letters to the FDA on the progress of the CAPA plan implementations until the CAPA is closed are also strongly advised and would be detailed in the initial response letter, i.e., the sponsor will provide the FDA with updates on the last Friday of each quarter until the response actions are closed. If there are any delays in the actions needed for the CAPAs, a justification and a description of what else was done as mitigation should be included in the follow-up. Once the CAPA is closed, documented evidence that the actions needed under the CAPA were completed is provided in the next update or after the last CAPA is closed.

Do not expect the FDA to respond to updates or even the final close-out letter that was submitted with supporting evidence when all the CAPAs have been addressed. There is no requirement for the FDA to reply to the sponsor. Be prepared to wait and see.

If the Agency is not satisfied with the response to the observations, it may send a warning letter, which indicates that either the explanation given for why the observation occurred or the remedial actions were inadequate. The warning letter specifies what still needs to be done to resolve the issue and will also indicate what regulatory action will be taken if compliance is not met. Warning letters are issued at any time to the most senior person at the sponsor and are considered a more significant regulatory action than the FDA 483. The Agency could also send an untitled letter to address violations that are not serious enough to invoke a warning letter but still may require remedial action. Sponsors are encouraged to have an open dialogue with the FDA and request clarification if necessary to resolve any misunderstandings and avoid any further regulatory actions. A more in-depth description of the FDA inspection process can be found at *Burgess, Cathy L., and Jarcho, Daniel G. FDA Inspection Process Chapter 21: Good Manufacturing Practices for Pharmaceuticals 2019.*

CONCLUSION

The results of BIMO inspections can mean the difference between an IP marketing application approval, the rejection of the application, or even a regulatory action against the sponsor. The development of the appropriate level of process, with a focus on critical quality attributes aligned with the regulations and audit preparedness, is a best practice to minimize the opportunity for serious inspection findings. Proper training on inspection readiness at an organizational level is essential to the success of the program. Rejected applications often mean further trials must be done or the program may be abandoned altogether, depending on the funding available. This is why many sponsors will hire experts in inspection readiness to increase their likelihood of positive outcomes from BIMO inspections in support of their marketing applications.

REFERENCES

1. *Freedom of Information Act (FOIA) Improvement Act of 2016. Public Law 114-185.* URL: https://www.justice.gov/oip/oip-summary-foia-improvement-act-2016
2. FDA. *Bioresearch Monitoring Program Information.* Food and Drug Administration. Retrieved 6 Feb 2024. URL: https://www.fda.gov/inspections-compliance-enforcement-and-criminal-investigations/fda-bioresearch-monitoring-information/bioresearch-monitoring-program-information.
3. FDA. *Bioresearch Monitoring Program (BIMO) Compliance Programs. Chapter 48 - Bioresearch Monitoring. 7348.810 Sponsors and Contract Research Organizations. Implemented* September 15, *2021.* Food and Drug Administration. Updated URL: https://www.fda.gov/inspections-compliance-enforcement-and-criminal-investigations/compliance-program-manual/bioresearch-monitoring-program-bimo-compliance-programs.
4. DOJ. *What is FOIA?* Department of Justice. Retrieved 6 Feb, 2024. URL: https://www.foia.gov/about.html.
5. FDA. *Freedom of Information. Food and Drug Administration.* Retrieved 6 Feb 2024. URL: https://www.fda.gov/regulatory-information/freedom-information.
6. ICH. ICH Harmonised Guideline. *General Considerations for Clinical Studies ICH E8(R1).* International Council for Harmonization of Technical Requirements for Pharmaceuticals for Human Use. 06 October2021.
7. ICH. *ICH Harmonised Guideline - Good Clinical Practice (GCP) E6(R3).* International Council for Harmonization of Technical Requirements for Pharmaceuticals for Human Use. 19 May 2023.
8. FDA. *Part 11, Electronic Records; Electronic Signatures - Scope and Application.* Food and Drug Administration. September 2003.
9. FDA. *Electronic Systems, Electronic Records, and Electronic Signatures in Clinical Investigations: Questions and Answers.* Food and Drug Administration. March 2023.

13 Regulations Relating to the Placebo Response in Clinical Research

Graham Bunn and Arthur Ooghe

INTRODUCTION TO THE PLACEBO RESPONSE

The placebo response, by definition, is the response measured in a group of patients undergoing a "dummy" treatment in a study. While often associated with the placebo effect – the improvement felt by a subject believing to receive an active treatment – it is actually the sum of influences on the course of the disease, except the pharmacologic effect of a drug [1]. These influences are numerous, including, for example, the natural progression of the disease, regression-to-the-mean, patient or investigator expectations, improvement in care due to better medical management, or the subjective role of certain diagnostic evaluations. These influences are specific to the subject's and study's contexts, which explains why the placebo response is also referred to as the contextual effect in the literature [2]. As these influences are not specific to any particular treatment, the contextual effect will contribute to the measured response in each of the treated groups in a clinical trial.

PLACEBO-CONTROLLED STUDY, THE GOLDEN STANDARD

The desire to discriminate between a patient's improvement due to these contextual influences and those obtained through the specific effect of a treatment implies the use of control groups in clinical studies [1]. While different types of comparators may be considered depending on the circumstances, the most common one is a treatment that appears identical to the tested treatment (in terms of color, weight, taste, etc.) but is inert, a placebo. The use of a placebo as a control group has several advantages. The main advantage is that it is the only comparator that allows for the evaluation of the absolute effect in terms of efficacy and safety of a new treatment [1]. As stated by the ICH, placebo control groups, combined with randomization and double blinding, controls for all potential influences on the actual or apparent course of the disease other than those arising from the pharmacologic action of the test drug. Furthermore, it is also the control requiring the smallest sample size to detect the effect of a treatment [1]. The main drawback of the placebo lies in the ethical questioning related to the acceptability of treating subjects with an inert substance. This can often be mitigated by adapting the study design: add-on studies, use of rescue treatment or early escapes, etc. However, the use of a placebo is not always possible, and other types of

DOI: 10.1201/9781003407010-13

controls must be considered: active comparator, untreated comparator, external comparator, etc. However, when using these other comparators, the contextual influences mentioned earlier remain either completely or partially:

- An active control will be subject to the same contextual influences, to which the specific pharmacologic effect of that treatment will be added. Recent meta-analyses have indeed shown that this contextual effect accounts for more than 50% on average in the overall response to treatment and explains a large part of the variability in this response [2–4].
- An untreated control will also be subject to influences such as the natural progression of the disease, regression-to-the-mean, etc.

The methods considered to apprehend the contextual effect, or placebo response, will therefore also be applicable to these other types of control, even without specifically considering a placebo group.

IMPACT OF THE PLACEBO RESPONSE AND INITIAL APPROACH TO OVERCOME IT

The impact of the contextual effect is directly related to its intrinsic source: the heterogeneity of the subject's profile. A greater heterogeneity among patients often leads to increased variability in contextual effects and consequently in responses across all groups. This heightened variability mechanically diminishes the effect size of a treatment, which is inversely proportional to variability, thus reducing assay sensitivity and study power. This phenomenon becomes particularly problematic as contextual effects and their variability have progressively increased over time [5,6], resulting in a rise in inconclusive clinical trials. The most straightforward approach to tackle this escalating variability is to increase sample sizes required to establish treatment efficacy. However, this approach raises concerns regarding the ethical implications of subjecting a larger number of individuals to ineffective or potentially unsafe substances. To mitigate the rise in sample sizes, which in turn escalates study costs and duration, alternative methods have been implemented to account for the increasing response variability in clinical trials.

One solution sometimes advocated is the utilization of a crossover study design. In the crossover design, each subject is randomized to a sequence of two or more treatments, thus serving as their own control for treatment comparisons. This feature initially makes this design appealing as the patient's context is no longer assumed to play a role in the difference between their responses to each treatment. The anticipated benefit of such a design is a significant reduction in the number of subjects required to achieve the desired study power. However, this reduction in required patients comes at the expense of study duration, which must be multiplied by the number of treatments evaluated at minimum. Furthermore, the ICH identifies numerous potential issues with this design, which could lead to the invalidation of study results [7]. The most significant concern is the understanding and management of carryover, which refers to the residual influence of treatments in subsequent treatment periods. This carryover issue raises questions about the extent to which efficacy and adverse events can be attributed to the evaluated treatment or those preceding it [7,8]. Lastly, subject dropout during the study complicates the analysis and interpretation of results. In summary, the ICH restricts this type of design to long-term studies of chronic and stable diseases, where dropout rates are expected to be very low, and sufficient knowledge exists to ensure an adequate washout period between each treatment.

PROGNOSTIC FACTORS AND COVARIATES

To directly address the contextual effect, it is crucial to understand the factors influencing it: **the prognostic factors**. The FDA defines a prognostic factor as a covariate measured at baseline that may be associated with the primary endpoint [9]. In other words, a prognostic factor can be any measure (demographic, psychosocial, medical, etc.) captured before the administration of any treatment in the clinical trial, capable of predicting an observable increase or decrease of the symptoms regardless of the treated group under consideration. These factors should not be confused with predictive factors that characterize symptom progression specific to a treatment or intervention. Understanding these influential elements enables the definition of useful methods to mitigate the impact of subjects' heterogeneity and their placebo response on assay sensitivity. For instance, training patients and/or clinical staff to reduce and standardize expectations or variability in symptom reporting is a solution frequently contemplated by sponsors [10]. Nevertheless, while these strategies have yielded some benefit to trials, the problem persists and other methods are often considered [11].

Another common method to leverage prognostic covariates is a randomization stratified for these factors. This stratification aims to promote balanced allocation within strata, with the potential benefit being more pronounced in small trials. Stratified randomization consequently diminishes the likelihood of imbalances that could favor one group [7]. The EMA highlights additional potential advantages, including a more efficient estimation of treatment effects, a greater credibility of study results, and the ability to ensure good distribution among groups of variables characterizing subgroup analyses [12]. However, it is not advisable to use more than 2 or 3 prognostic factors for stratification. This limitation notably reduces the likelihood of achieving adequate balance and poses logistical challenges [7].

While regulatory agencies do not define which prognostic factors are of interest, they do have dedicated guidance on methods that leverage them. Two major options in particular are discussed: enriching the study population based on a patient characteristic and/or adjusting the statistical analysis of the study for this characteristic.

ENRICHMENT: DECREASING HETEROGENEITY AT THE COST OF GENERALIZABILITY

Enrichment refers to the prospective utilization of any patient characteristic to select a study population in which the detection of a potential drug effect is more likely than in an unselected population. This particular point has been discussed by the FDA in guidance initially published in draft form in 2012 and finalized in 2019.

This guidance primarily focuses on the impact of such methods on the efficacy analyses of a treatment [13]. However, it draws parallels with the possibility of implementing equivalent procedures for safety considerations as well. According to the FDA, enrichment methods can be distinguished based on three different objectives:

1. Strategies aimed at reducing patient heterogeneity.
2. Those targeting patients having a disease-related endpoint event (for event-driven studies) or a substantial worsening in condition (for continuous measurement endpoints).
3. Predictive strategies aimed at patients more likely to benefit from the treatment under study.

The first category thus involves leveraging knowledge of prognostic patient characteristics to reduce the observed variability in the placebo response. Enrichment can be based on either a binary characteristic (e.g., sex, presence of genetic marker(s), a concomitant illness) or a continuous one (e.g., age, blood pressure (BP), body mass index (BMI)). However, the second case requires categorizing the variable. As emphasized in this guidance, reducing variability through this strategy enhances assay sensitivity and increases study power. However, the use of enrichment raises two questions: the validity of the study results and their generalizability. According to the FDA, enrichment must be explicitly described and set in the protocol before the study initiation. If this condition is met, enrichment does not compromise the statistical validity of the trials, or the meaningfulness of the conclusions reached for the population actually studied. However, the generalizability and applicability of these results to the population excluded from the study are generally not automatic and must be explicitly discussed in the protocol and study report, along with fully detailing the rationale for the design, the specific enrichment maneuvers, and their effects on the interpretation of results. Enrichment may also specifically go against the FDA's important guidance on inclusivity for clinical trials which is a key driver within the whole industry right now [14].

ADJUSTMENT: A LOW-RISK METHOD TO INCREASE ASSAY SENSITIVITY

Adjustment is another way to leverage prognostic factors to enhance assay sensitivity. Adjusted analysis refers to a statistical technique used to assess an outcome while considering the influence of prognostic covariates. Unlike enrichment, this method does not involve reducing the targeted study population nor changing the study design. While adjustment for prognostic covariates was already discussed in ICH E9 [7], it has subsequently been addressed in specific guidelines, first by the EMA in 2015 [12], and then by the FDA, whose final guidance was released in 2023 [9]. The latter, being the most recent, likely offers the most comprehensive insights into this topic.

The general recommendations of the FDA can be summarized easily. An analysis of an efficacy endpoint can be unadjusted. However, an analysis adjusted for baseline covariates can lead to a reduction in the confidence interval of the treatment effect estimation and a more powerful test. Moreover, the adjustment can be done with minimal impact on bias or the Type I error rate, as long as they are measured at baseline and predefined in the protocol. These covariates can be derived from the scientific literature or defined and/or constructed based on previous studies, emphasizing the recent interest in developing more complex prognostic models (see e.g., [15]). The greater the association between these covariates and the endpoint, the greater the gain in precision will be. However, even an adjusted analysis for covariates that are ultimately not associated with the response remains valid. Finally, multiple prognostic covariates can be used to adjust an analysis, but ideally, their number should remain small compared to the sample size. These covariates can be correlated with each other, but the benefit will generally be greater when their correlation is low. Furthermore, for the vast majority of outcomes and associated models used in current clinical studies, adjusted analysis remains valid even if the model is misspecified or if the association between covariates and the endpoint is weaker than expected, provided certain rules in model definition are respected.

According to this guidance, the FDA strongly recommends the use of adjustment covariates to improve the precision of treatment effect estimation.

CONCLUSION

The placebo response, or contextual effect, poses a significant obstacle to the precise estimation of treatment effects in clinical studies. The initial response to this issue by sponsors and regulatory agencies has been to utilize a control group, typically a placebo, along with double-blinding randomization [1]. While this approach effectively segregates the portion of response attributable to the study treatment from other effects, it does not address the problem of patient heterogeneity and the considerable variability in their contextual effects. This variability represents therefore the primary challenge in managing the placebo response, as it tends to diminish assay sensitivity.

Sponsors of clinical trials have traditionally implemented various methods to control or mitigate the impact of the placebo response. These efforts typically focus on:

- Increasing the size of the study patient population
- Exploring alternative study designs such as crossover trials
- Minimizing the amplification of patient expectations, either through factors inherent to the clinical trial design or through training of site personnel
- Reducing variation or errors in patient or physician/rater reporting of outcomes through training programs.

While these strategies have shown some effectiveness in trials, the issue persists, with some reports suggesting that the placebo response and its variability are actually on the rise over time, particularly in areas such as pain management [5] and psychiatry [6].

To effectively mitigate the placebo response, it is essential to understand and model it comprehensively. This requires a clear definition of prognostic factors. Understanding these factors associated with contextual response allows for direct intervention in the variability of the response observed in clinical trial. Regulatory agencies recognize the importance of this and are actively discussing various methodologies in their guidance documents. Currently, three main categories of methods are under consideration:

- Stratified randomization based on prognostic factors
- Enrichment strategies aimed at reducing heterogeneity
- Adjustment of statistical analyses to account for prognostic factors measured at baseline.

Stratified randomization enhances the efficacy of treatment effect estimators by ensuring a proper balance of prognostic factors used for stratification. However, it does not alleviate the heterogeneity of the measured response within each group and can only be performed for a limited number of factors due to logistical constraints. On the other hand, enrichment reduces patient heterogeneity and consequently the variability of the observed response. This enhances the assay sensitivity of the statistical analysis, which remains valid as long as the enrichment is pre-defined in the protocol and based on a baseline measure. Unfortunately, enrichment raises concerns regarding the generalizability of results to patients excluded from the study and increases the duration and cost of patient screening. Finally, adjustment corrects imbalances between groups, like the stratification. However, it also accounts for the effect of the considered prognostic factors on response variability, thereby augmenting assay sensitivity. If the adjustment factors are baseline and predefined, this generally poses no risk to analysis validity. Moreover, this has a beneficial effect on analysis precision as long as the prognostic factors adequately explain differences in response between patients. Adjustment for prognostic variables can thus be seen as a low-risk solution, justifying the FDA's positive stance on it as well as its widespread endorsement in specialized scientific literature [16,17].

BIBLIOGRAPHY

[1] ICH, "E10- Choice of control group and related issues in clinical trials," *ICH Harmonised Guideline,* 2000.

[2] K. Zou, J. Wong, N. Abdullah, X. Chen, T. Smith, M. Doherty and W. Zhang, "Examination of overall treatment effect and the proportion attributable to contextual effect in osteoarthritis: meta-analysis of randomised controlled trials," *Annals of the Rheumatic Diseases,* vol. 75, pp. 1964–1970, 2016.

[3] S. H. Hafliðadóttir, C. B. Juhl, S. M. Nielsen, M. Henriksen, I. Harris, H. Bliddal and R. Christensen, "Placebo response and effects in randomized clinical trials: protocol for a meta-analysis with focus on contextual effects," *Trials,* vol. 22, no. 493, pp. 1–15, 2021.

[4] H. Walach, C. Sadaghiani, C. Dehm and D. Bierman, "The therapeutic effect of clinical trials: understanding placebo response rates in clinical trials - a secondary analysis," *BMC Medical Research Methodology,* vol. 5, pp. 1–12, 2005.

[5] A. H. Tuttle, S. Tohyama, T. Ramsay, J. Kimmelman, P. Schweinhardt, G. J. Bennett and J. S. Mogil, "Increasing placebo responses over time in U.S. clinical trials of neuropathic pain," *Pain,* vol. 156, no. 12, pp. 2616–2626, 2015.

[6] M. Gopalakrishnan, H. Zhu, T. R. Farchione, M. Mathis, M. Mehta, R. Uppoor and I. Younis, "The trend of increasing placebo response and decreasing treatment effect in schizophrenia trials continues: an update from the US Food and Drug Administration," *The Journal of Clinical Psychiatry,* vol. 81, no. 2, p. 14594, 2020.

[7] ICH, "E9- Statistical principles for clinical trials," *ICH Harmonised Guideline,* 1998.

[8] ICH, "E4- Dose response information to support drug registration step," *ICH Harmonised Guideline,* 1994.

[9] FDA, "Adjusting for covariates in randomized clinical trials for drugs and biological products," 2023.

[10] R. R. Edwards, R. H. Dworkin, D. C. Turk, M. S. Angst, R. Dionne, R. Freeman, P. Hansson, S. Haroutounian, L. Arendt-Nielsen, N. Attal, R. Baron, J. Brell, S. Bujanover, L. B. Burke, and D. Carr, "Patient phenotyping in clinical trials of chronic pain treatments: IMMPACT recommendations," *Pain Reports,* vol. 157, no. 9, pp. 1851–1871, 2016.

[11] E. A. Smith, W. P. Horan, D. Demolle, P. Schueler, D.-J. Fu, A. E. Anderson and J. Geraci, "Using artificial intelligence-based methods to address the placebo response in clinical trials," *Innovations in Clinical Neuroscience,* vol. 19, no. 1–3, pp. 60–70, 2022.

[12] EMA, *Guideline on adjustment for baseline covariates in clinical trials.* London: European Medicines Agency, 2015.

[13] FDA, "Enrichment strategies for clinical trials to support determination of effectiveness of human drugs and biological products guidance for industry," *Guidance for Industry,* 2019.

[14] FDA, "Enhancing the diversity of clinical trial populations - eligibility criteria, enrollment practices, and trial designs guidance for industry," *FDA-2019-D-1264,* 2020.

[15] S. Branders, A. Pereira, G. Bernard, M. Ernst, J. Dananberg and A. Albert, "Leveraging historical data to optimize the number of covariates and their explained variance in the analysis of randomized clinical trials.," *Statistical Methods in Medical Research,* vol. 31, no. 2, pp. 240–252, 2022.

[16] B. C. Kahan, V. Jairath, C. J. Doré and T. P. Morris, "The risks and rewards of covariate adjustment in randomized trials: An assessment of 12 outcomes from 8 studies.," *Trials,* vol. 15, no. 139, pp. 1–7, 2014.

[17] D. J. Langford, S. Sharma, M. P. McDermott, A. Beeram, S. Besherat, F. O. France, R. Mark and M. Park, "Covariate Adjustment in Chronic Pain Trials: An Oft-Missed Opportunity," *The Journal of Pain,* vol. 24, no. 9, pp. 1555–1569, 2023.

Index

Note: **Bold** page numbers refer to tables; *italic* page numbers refer to figures and page numbers followed by "n" denote endnotes.

For Product Safety Concerns and Information please contact our EU representative GPSR@taylorandfrancis.com
Taylor & Francis Verlag GmbH, Kaufingerstraße 24, 80331 München, Germany

www.ingramcontent.com/pod-product-compliance
Lightning Source LLC
LaVergne TN
LVHW010602110826
845149LV00003B/744

* 9 7 8 1 0 3 2 5 2 5 2 5 9 *